Hungry Girl

SIMPLY
6

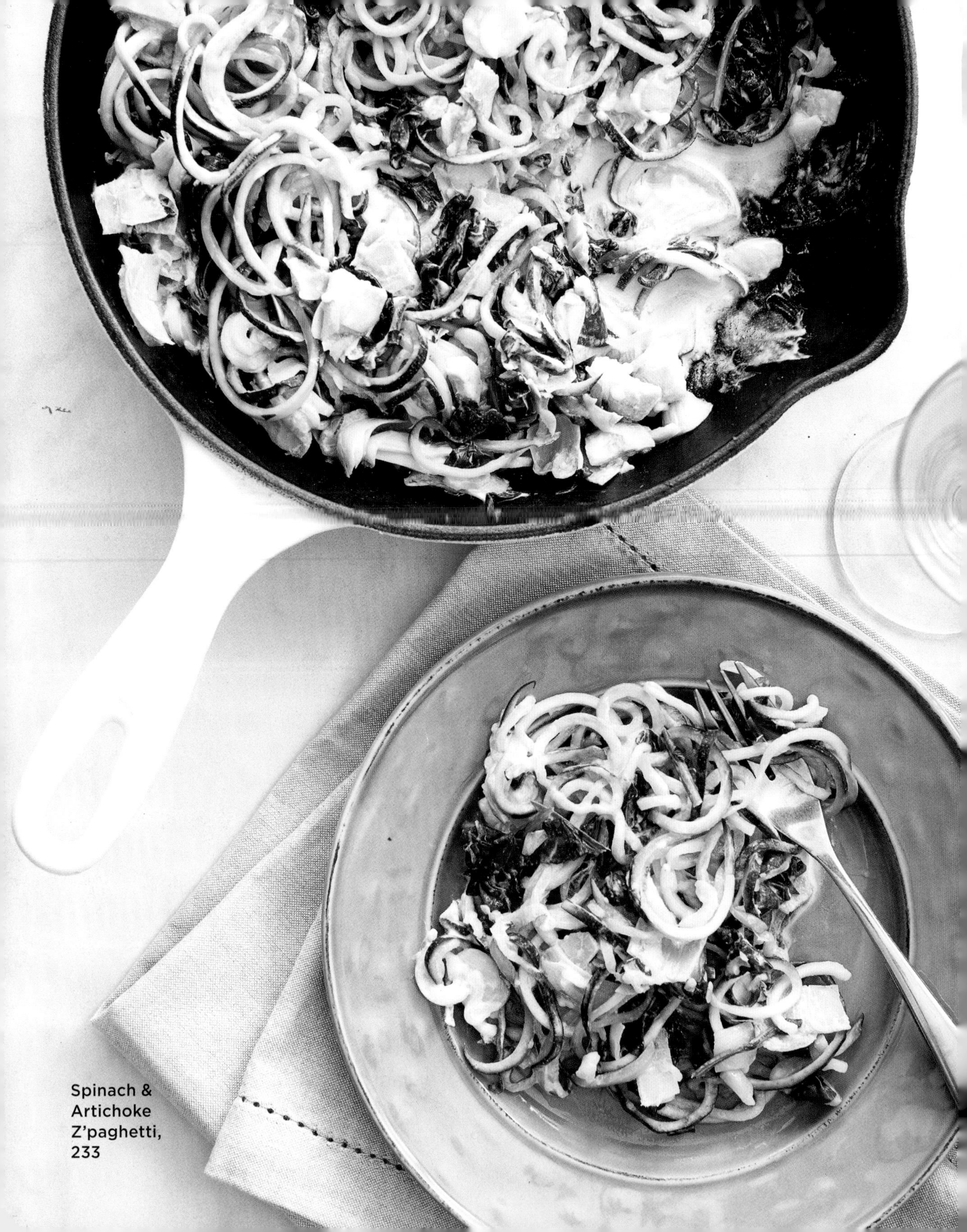

Spinach &
Artichoke
Z'paghetti,
233

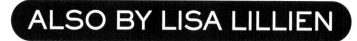

ALSO BY LISA LILLIEN

HUNGRY GIRL:
Recipes and Survival Strategies for Guilt-Free Eating in the Real World

HUNGRY GIRL 200 UNDER 200:
200 Recipes Under 200 Calories

HUNGRY GIRL 1-2-3:
The Easiest, Most Delicious, Guilt-Free Recipes on the Planet

HUNGRY GIRL HAPPY HOUR:
75 Recipes for Amazingly Fantastic Guilt-Free Cocktails & Party Foods

HUNGRY GIRL 300 UNDER 300:
300 Breakfast, Lunch & Dinner Dishes Under 300 Calories

HUNGRY GIRL SUPERMARKET SURVIVAL:
Aisle by Aisle, HG-Style!

HUNGRY GIRL TO THE MAX!
The Ultimate Guilt-Free Cookbook

HUNGRY GIRL 200 UNDER 200 JUST DESSERTS:
200 Recipes Under 200 Calories

THE HUNGRY GIRL DIET

THE HUNGRY GIRL DIET COOKBOOK:
Healthy Recipes for Mix-n-Match Meals & Snacks

HUNGRY GIRL CLEAN & HUNGRY:
Easy All-Natural Recipes for Healthy Eating in the Real World

HUNGRY GIRL CLEAN & HUNGRY OBSESSED!
All-Natural Recipes for the Foods You Can't Live Without

HUNGRY GIRL: THE OFFICIAL SURVIVAL GUIDES:
Tips & Tricks for Guilt-Free Eating
(audio book)

HUNGRY GIRL CHEW THE RIGHT THING:
Supreme Makeovers for 50 Foods You Crave
(recipe cards)

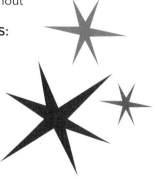

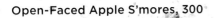

Open-Faced Apple S'mores, 300

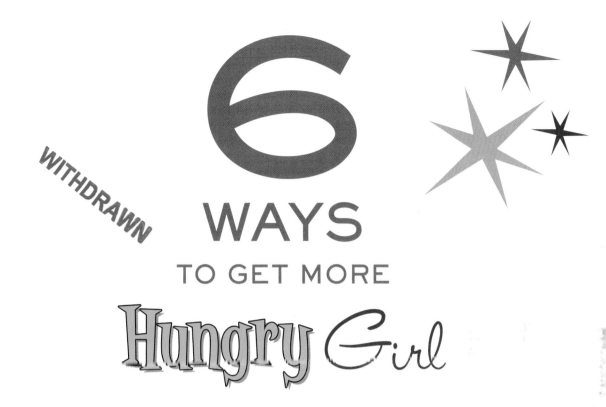

6 WAYS TO GET MORE Hungry Girl

WITHDRAWN

For the latest recipes, food finds, go-to guides, behind-the-scenes fun, and more . . .

✉ Sign up for **FREE daily emails** at hungry-girl.com

f Follow **Lisa on Facebook** at facebook.com/hungrygirl

👥 Join the **Hungry Girl Community: What's Chewin'?** on Facebook

📷 Follow **Lisa on Instagram**. Handle: hungrygirl

📌 Check out **Hungry Girl on Pinterest** at pinterest.com/hungrygirl

🎧 Listen to the *Hungry Girl: Chew the Right Thing!* podcast at hungry-girl.com/podcast

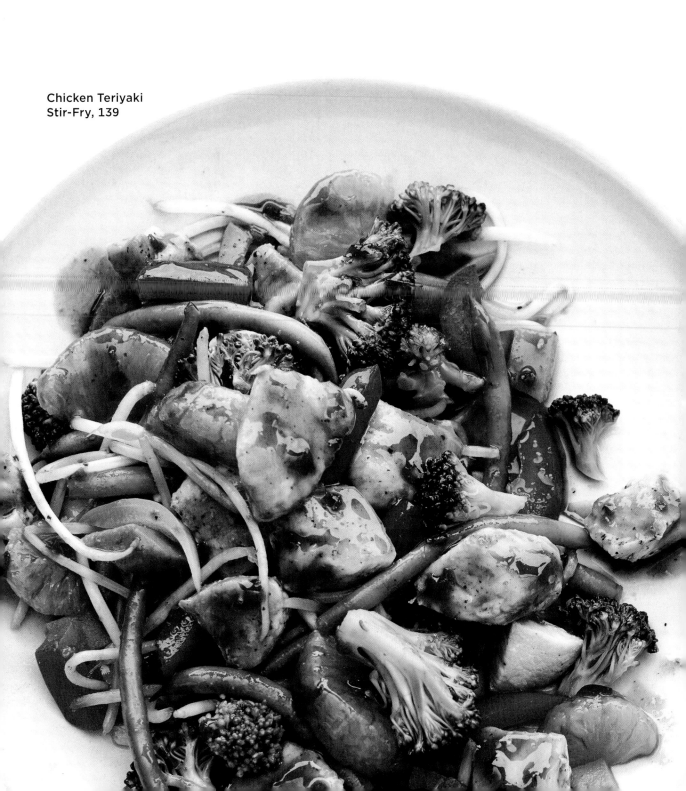

Chicken Teriyaki
Stir-Fry, 139

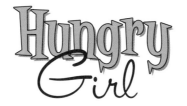

SIMPLY 6

ALL-NATURAL RECIPES WITH 6 INGREDIENTS OR LESS

LISA LILLIEN

St. Martin's Griffin ✎ New York

HUNGRY GIRL SIMPLY 6: All-Natural Recipes with 6 Ingredients or Less. Copyright © 2019 by Hungry Girl, Inc. All rights reserved. Printed in the United States of America. For information, address St. Martin's Press, 175 Fifth Avenue, New York, N.Y. 10010.

www.stmartins.com

Cover design by Ralph Fowler
Book design by Ralph Fowler
Illustrations by Jack Pullan
Food styling by Marian Cooper Cairns
Food photography by Jennifer Davick

The Library of Congress Cataloging-in-Publication Data is available upon request.

ISBN 978-1-250-15452-1 (trade paperback)
ISBN 978-1-250-15453-8 (ebook)

Our books may be purchased in bulk for promotional, educational, or business use. Please contact your local bookseller or the Macmillan Corporate and Premium Sales Department at 1-800-221-7945, extension 5442, or by email at MacmillanSpecialMarkets@macmillan.com.

First Edition: March 2019

10 9 8 7 6 5 4 3 2 1

This book is dedicated to
all the people out there who don't like
recipes with long ingredient lists.

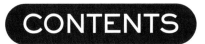

CONTENTS

1

SIMPLY EGGS

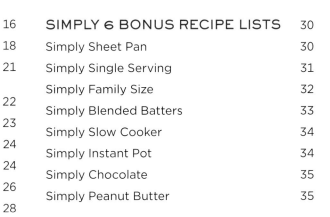

Broc 'n Cheddar Crustless Quiche, 50

2
SIMPLY OATS

3
SIMPLY CHICKEN

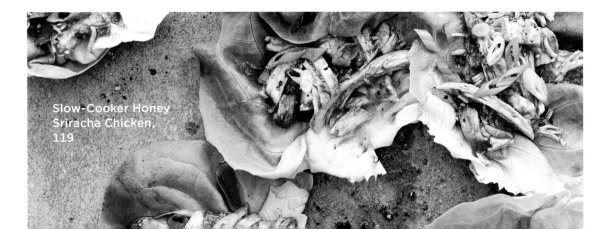

Slow-Cooker Honey
Sriracha Chicken,
119

4

SIMPLY BEEF (& PORK)

5

SIMPLY SEAFOOD

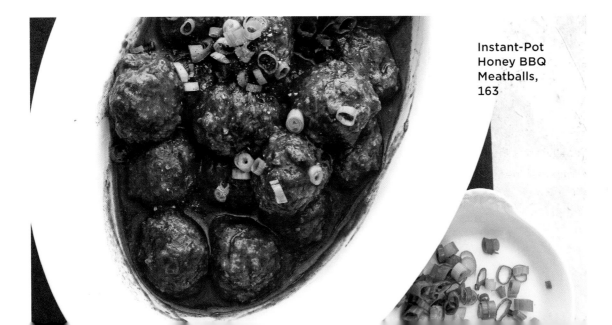

Instant-Pot Honey BBQ Meatballs, 163

6
SIMPLY VEGGIE

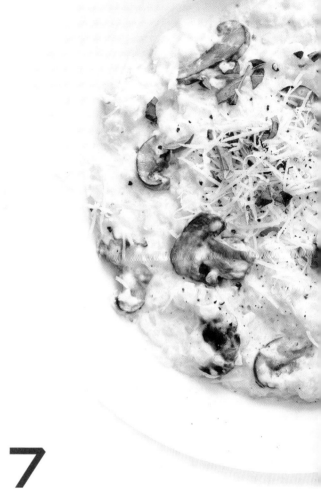

Mushroom
Faux-sotto, 252

7
SIMPLY DOUGH

8
SIMPLY FRUIT

9
SIMPLY MORE . . . SWEETS!

Scoopable
Upside-Down
Blueberry Pie,
295

10
SIMPLY SIMPLE: TIPS & TRICKS

Chocolate Cake in a Mug, 347

ACKNOWLEDGMENTS

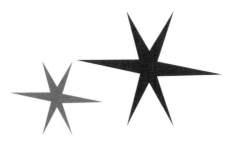

Jamie Goldberg——After over a dozen years, you still give 110 percent to all things Hungry Girl! Thank you for being a constant source of unwavering support, a true creative collaborator, and the glue that holds our team together! You are the BEST!

GINORMOUS thank-yous go out to the incomparable HG book team——you all ROCK and are so appreciated!

Lynn Bettencourt
Dana DeRuyck
Erin Norcross
Katie Killeavy
Lydia Oxenham
Julie Leonard

Special thanks to the following HGers for all they do . . .

Peggy Mansfield
Gina Muscato
Mike Sherry
Cindy Sloop
Olga Gatica

Shrimp Scampi Z'paghetti, 203

Bigtime thanks as well to the extended Hungry Girl family . . .

John Vaccaro
Neeti Madan
Jennifer Enderlin
John Karle
Anne Marie Tallberg
Brant Janeway
Jordan Hanley
Elizabeth Catalano
Rachel Diebel
James Sinclair
Cheryl Mamaril
Tracey Guest
Bill Stankey
Tom Fineman
Steve Younger
Jeff Becker
Susan Garcia
Ruby Magsambol
Lauren Lillien

Special shout-outs to these creative folks . . .

Ralph Fowler
Jennifer Davick
Marian Cooper Cairns
Jack Pullan

And, as always, endless gratitude and love to my incredible husband and family . . .

Daniel Schneider
Florence and Maurice Lillien
Meri Lillien
Jay Lillien
Lolly and Jordan

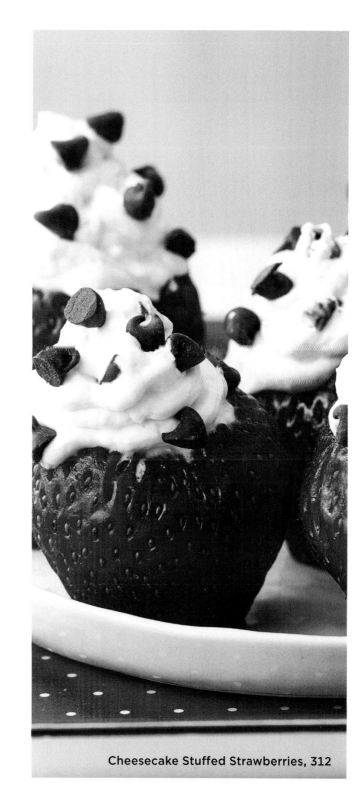

Cheesecake Stuffed Strawberries, 312

Hi,

Lisa here! I can hardly believe it, but *Simply 6* is my THIRTEENTH Hungry Girl book. And lucky you, because it's the one with the EASIEST (and quite possibly the most delicious) recipes of all! **Here are six simple things you might not know about me . . . and about this book!**

1. I LOVE simple and easy recipes.

When I started sending Hungry Girl daily emails back in 2004, my goal was to create ridiculously easy and delicious recipes. Many of the early recipes were so simple that they were actually more like food assembly! It's always been a goal of mine to make better-for-you recipes that anyone (and I mean ANYONE!) can make. I think this book delivers in spades, and you're going to LOVE it . . .

2. FUN FACT: When I was younger, I would flip through cookbook recipes that looked appealing . . .

. . . then immediately put the book down because it featured weird ingredients or complicated instructions. I simply did not want to deal with anything challenging in the kitchen. (I still don't!) My recipes are super easy and make people who *think* they're kitchen klutzes feel like chefs. It makes the Hungry Girl brand relatable and attainable, and I'm really proud of that!

3. After 12 books, I knew it was finally time to put together a collection of fast and easy recipes with very few ingredients for the audience.

It's what everyone has been asking for! Every recipe in this cookbook has six (or fewer!) main ingredients. You'll find future classics, family favorites, and simplified versions of dishes you could never imagine making with only six ingredients.

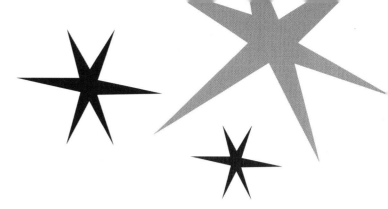

4. Sometimes, I play favorites.

In this book, my favorite recipe may be the Eggplant Lasagna (page 167) . . . or it could be Instant-Pot Honey BBQ Meatballs (page 163) . . . or possibly the Greek Z'paghetti (page 237) or the Garlic Knots (page 280) . . . AHHHH! I love too many to pick just one.

5. I'm an information junkie, so here are some important stats for you.

Every recipe in this book has less than 375 calories per serving. More than half of them will take you 30 minutes or less to prepare . . . and two dozen of those take 15 minutes or less! A whopping 18 of the recipes require NO COOKING AT ALL, 95 are GLUTEN-FREE, 91 of them are VEGETARIAN, and 147 are 100% DELICIOUS (that's ALL of them, don't worry!).

6. I truly couldn't be more excited about bringing these recipes to you.

They're incredibly delicious and easy, and I can't wait for you to try them. Once you do, please let me know how you like 'em! I always love to hear from you, and I welcome all feedback, so please don't be shy. Send me an email at suggest@ hungry-girl.com. I read every single email!

Happy chewing!!!

Lisa :)

Bageled Eggs, 62

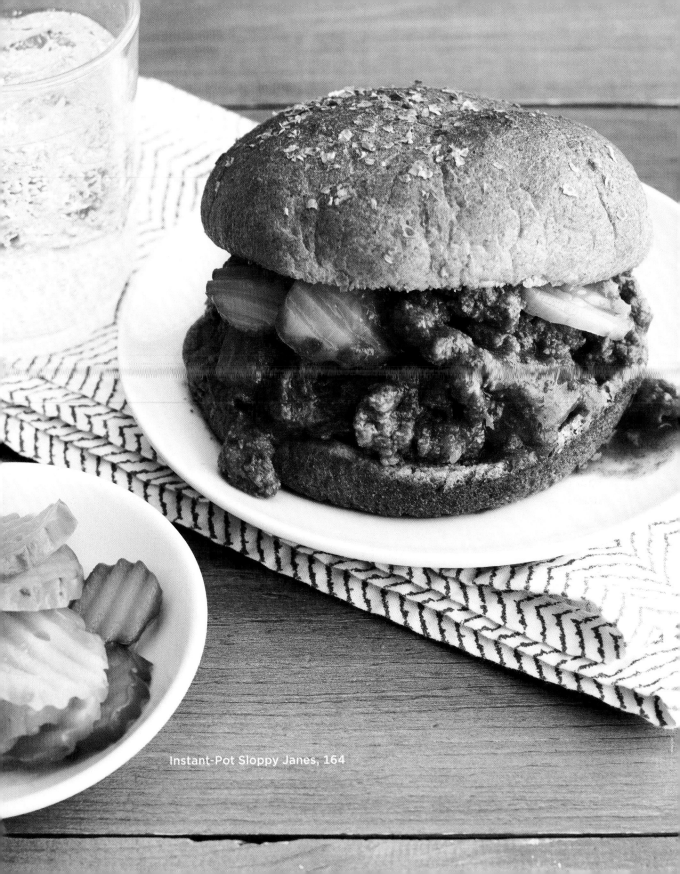

Instant-Pot Sloppy Janes, 164

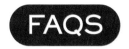

FAQS

What does Simply 6 mean?

It simply means each of these recipes calls for SIX (or fewer!) main ingredients.

What doesn't count as a main ingredient? Water, ice, basic seasonings, and serving suggestions. Look for the "Extra, Extra!" callouts to identify any optional ingredients. You'll also see the occasional herb garnish in photos. Feel free to garnish your dishes any way you like . . . or not at all!

Also, the ingredients called for in this book are SUPER-SIMPLE supermarket staples. No pomegranate molasses or organic rose water here!

What makes these recipes all natural?

The recipes in this book feature lots of "whole" natural ingredients: lean protein, fruits & veggies, eggs, oats, etc. When it comes to other foods called for in the recipes—like cheese, condiments, and canned goods—each and every one of those is readily available without any artificial ingredients. When in doubt, look for all-natural brands, read the product's ingredient list, or just stick to a natural food store.

Are these recipes good for diabetics or people on a low-sodium diet?

Remember, I'm not a nutrition professional. (I'm just hungry!) So I don't offer medical advice related to any dietary conditions. What I can (and WILL!) do, however, is provide full nutritional info for every recipe. The information is carefully calculated and confirmed using reliable databases and countless product labels. This way, you can review each recipe and its nutritional info to determine what works for YOU.

Generally, my recipes are low in added sugar and starchy carbs, and the sodium per serving tops out at 875mg. (For most recipes, the sodium is much lower. Also, there's a sodium-saving guide on page 359.) And I've heard from MANY fans with different dietary requirements that they can make a simple swap here and there so the recipes meet their needs.

Where can I find the WW (formerly Weight Watchers) points values?

I'm a big fan of WW, and I know many of you are too! That's why my team and I always calculate the points value for each Hungry Girl recipe. At WW's request—and because the points system has been known to change over time—these values are provided on the Hungry Girl website as opposed to printed in this book . . .

Visit hungry-girl.com/simply6 for the WW points values*!

*The Freestyle™ SmartPoints® values for these recipes were calculated by Hungry Girl
and are not an endorsement or approval of the recipe or its developer by
WW International, Inc., the owner of the SmartPoints® trademark.

RECIPE GUIDE

Craving gluten-free, vegetarian, or super-speedy recipes? Look for these symbols next to each recipe . . . or just peruse the listings on the following pages.

And don't miss the BONUS recipe lists starting on page 30 . . . Simply Slow Cooker, Simply Family Size, and more!

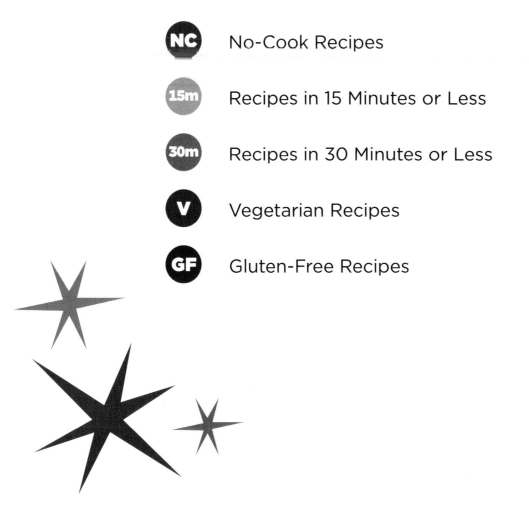

NC No-Cook Recipes

15m Recipes in 15 Minutes or Less

30m Recipes in 30 Minutes or Less

V Vegetarian Recipes

GF Gluten-Free Recipes

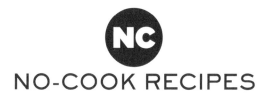

NO-COOK RECIPES

Step away from the stove, oven, and microwave. These recipes are keeping it cool with prep and chill/freeze times only.

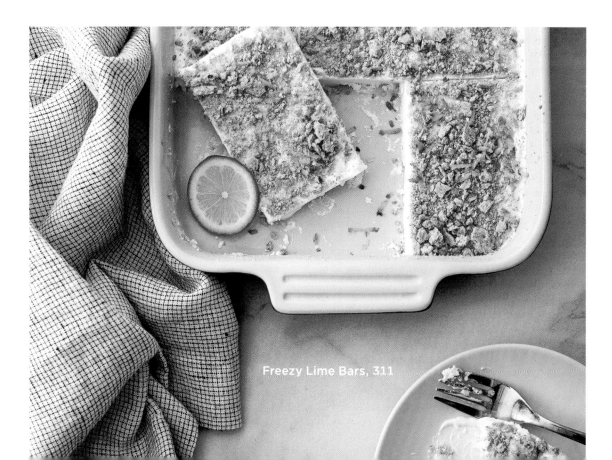

Freezy Lime Bars, 311

RECIPES IN 15 MINUTES OR LESS

From start to finish, each of these recipes will be
ready in no more than 15 minutes!

RECIPES IN 30 MINUTES OR LESS

Combined with the recipes in the list above, you're looking at more than
HALF the recipes in the book that can be made in a half hour or less. Wow!

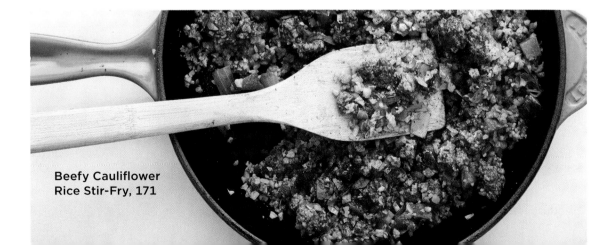

Beefy Cauliflower Rice Stir-Fry, 171

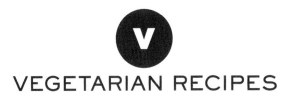

VEGETARIAN RECIPES

These recipes are made without red meat, poultry, seafood, or any ingredients made with those foods, like chicken broth. (They may contain dairy and/or egg but can usually be made vegan with some tweaks.)

HG HEADS UP

Some brands add animal-derived ingredients to otherwise vegetarian-friendly foods. For example, yogurt may contain gelatin. Check those labels!

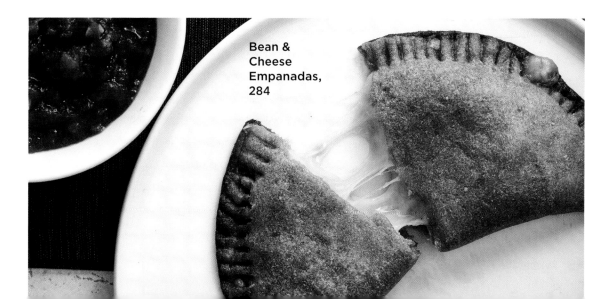

Bean & Cheese Empanadas, 284

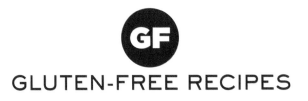

GLUTEN-FREE RECIPES

All the ingredients in these recipes are naturally gluten-free. Yes!

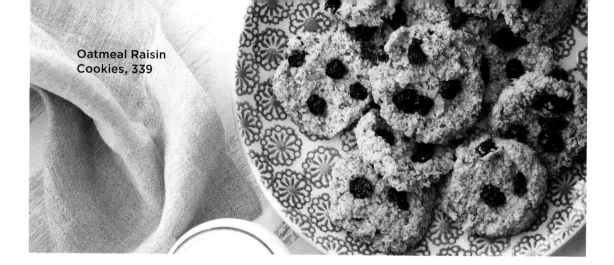
Oatmeal Raisin
Cookies, 339

HG HEADS UP

Naturally gluten-free foods may contain a hint of gluten due to cross contamination. For example, some oat companies warn of equipment shared with gluten-containing grains. If you're sensitive to gluten, read labels carefully.

SIMPLY 6 BONUS RECIPE LISTS

Did you find the recipe guide helpful? Good! Because I've got more roundups to make your life easier . . .

SIMPLY SHEET PAN

Cooking up something healthy and delicious is so easy when all it takes is a baking sheet!

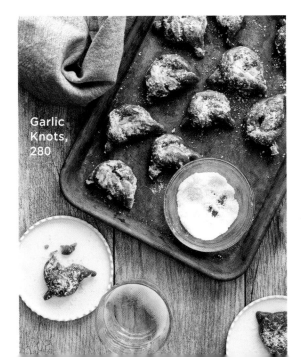

Garlic Knots, 280

SIMPLY SINGLE SERVING

Not in the mood for leftovers? These recipes for one will save the day . . .

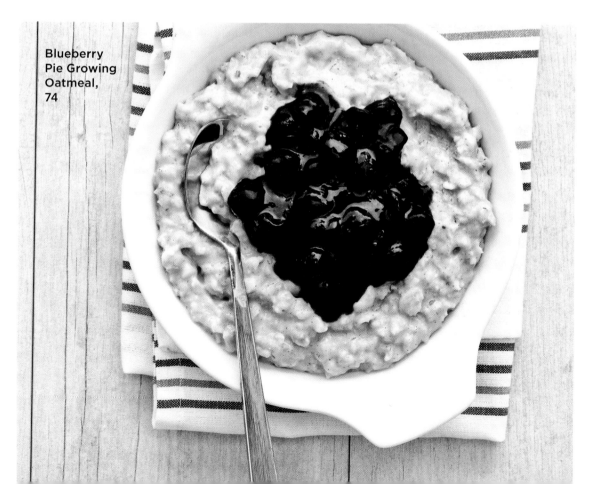

Blueberry Pie Growing Oatmeal, 74

SIMPLY FAMILY SIZE

Each of these recipes serves four or more! Perfect for feeding the family or whipping up multiple make-ahead meals (more about those on page 366!).

SIMPLY BLENDED BATTERS

Forget using multiple bowls and a whisk, plus exhausting your mixing arm . . . These easy recipes make use of your blender. So simple!

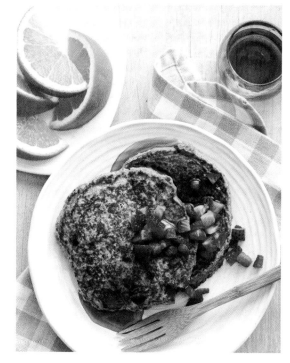

Strawberry Banana Blender Pancakes, 88

SIMPLY SLOW COOKER

No slow cooker? No problem! Check out page 360 to learn
how to make these recipes in a pot on your stove!

SIMPLY INSTANT POT

The trendy countertop gadget makes speedy meals a
breeze! Page 361 has all the need-to-know info, including
how make these recipes without an Instant Pot . . .

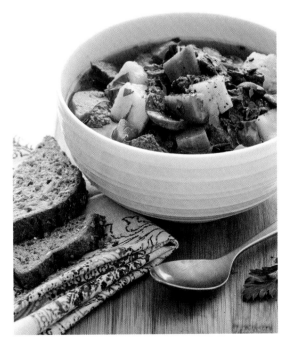

**Instant-Pot Chunky
Beef Soup, 183**

SIMPLY CHOCOLATE

You'll find all the chocolatey creations here!

SIMPLY PEANUT BUTTER

Attention PB lovers . . . You'll likely need to bookmark this list!

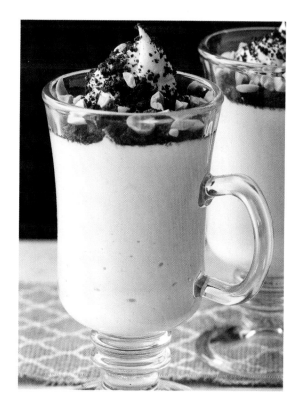

Peanut Butter Pie in a Mug, 352

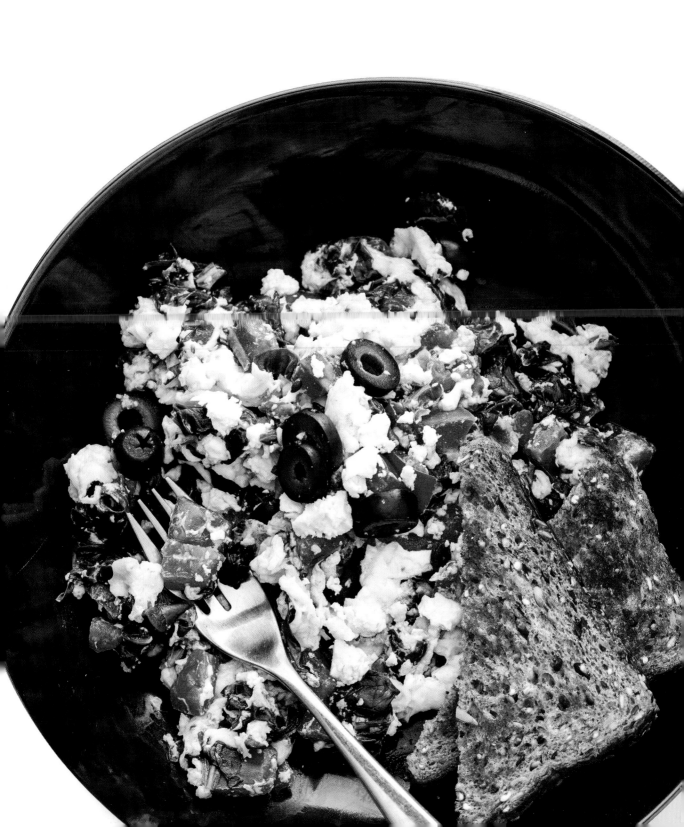

1

SIMPLY EGGS

Eggs are a breakfast staple in my world. They're protein packed and so satisfying! These recipes are creative, flavorful, and easy to make.

CHICKEN SAUSAGE EGG MUG

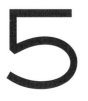 **Entire recipe:** 263 calories, 9.5g total fat (4.5g sat fat), 704mg sodium, 12g carbs, 2g fiber, 5g sugars, 30.5g protein

5

½ cup chopped **asparagus**
¼ cup chopped **onion**
¾ cup (about 6 large) **egg whites** or **fat-free liquid egg substitute**
2 tablespoons **light/reduced-fat cream cheese**
1½ ounces (about ½ link) **fully cooked chicken sausage**, chopped

seasonings:
⅛ teaspoon garlic powder

You'll need: large microwave-safe mug, nonstick spray

Prep: 5 minutes
Cook: 10 minutes

1. In a large microwave-safe mug sprayed with nonstick spray, combine asparagus, onion, and 1 tablespoon water. Cover, and microwave for 1½ minutes, or until softened.

2. Drain water, and blot away excess moisture. Add egg and garlic powder, and stir. Microwave for 2 minutes.

3. Stir in cream cheese and chopped sausage. Microwave for 2 minutes, or until set.

MAKES 1 SERVING

SURVEY SAYS . . .

59% of Hungry Girl fans say ketchup has no place on eggs. What do YOU think?

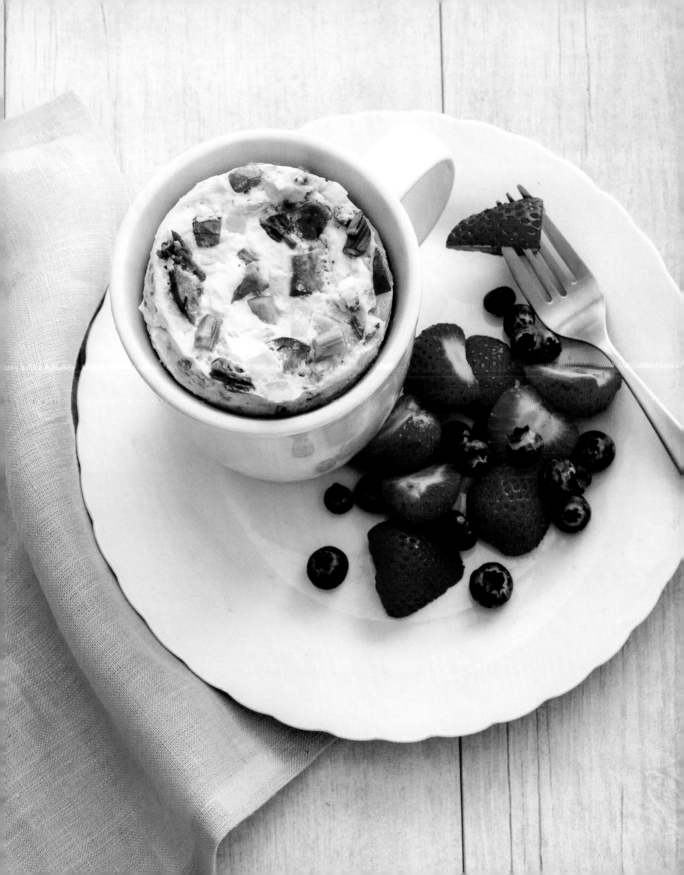

Build Your Own Egg Mug

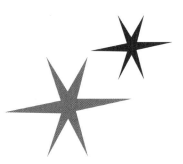

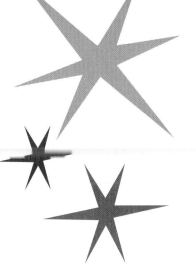

Making egg scrambles in the microwave is life changing. You get a hot & hearty breakfast (or snack) in minutes, and there are no skillets or spatulas to clean! Don't limit yourself to the recipe on the previous page . . . Create your own combinations!

How To

Step 1: Spray a large microwave-safe mug with nonstick spray. The bigger the better . . . Eggs puff up as they cook!

Step 2: Throw in some diced veggies and a bit of water. Microwave for 1 minute, or until softened.

Step 3: Blot away excess moisture. Add egg whites or egg substitute, sprinkle with some seasonings, and mix it up.

Step 4: Microwave for 1 minute. (You're almost done!)

Step 5: Add your mix-ins, and microwave for 30 seconds, or until egg is fully cooked and mix-ins are hot.

Step 6: Top it off!

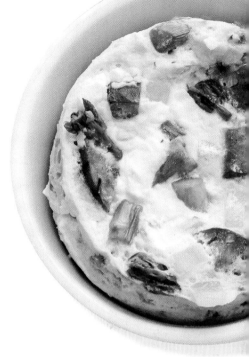

Mix 'n Match Ingredients

Feel free to go rogue, but these are some of my favorites!

Veggies

onion • bell pepper • spinach • mushrooms • tomatoes • asparagus • zucchini • frozen corn • broccoli cole slaw

Mix-Ins

shredded reduced-fat cheese (cheddar, Mexican-blend, or mozzarella) • feta cheese • reduced-fat/light cream cheese • fully cooked sausage (chicken, turkey, or meatless) • shredded chicken breast • crumbled bacon (turkey or center-cut) • chopped lean deli meat

Toppings

salsa • ketchup • avocado • light sour cream • scallions • basil • cilantro • hot sauce • fat-free Greek yogurt

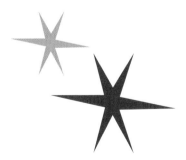

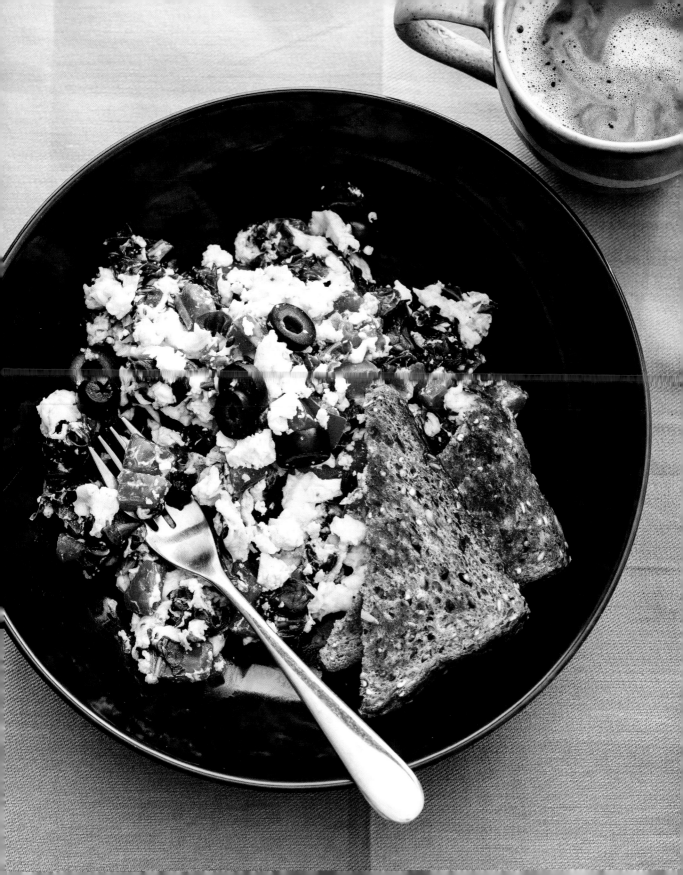

MEDITERRANEAN SCRAMBLE

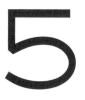 **Entire recipe:** 199 calories, 5.5g total fat (2.5g sat fat), 682mg sodium, 10.5g carbs, 3g fiber, 3g sugars, 25g protein

5

¾ cup (about 6 large) **egg whites** or **fat-free liquid egg substitute**
3 cups chopped **spinach**
½ cup seeded and chopped **tomato**
2 tablespoons sliced **olives**
2 tablespoons crumbled **feta cheese**

seasonings:
⅛ teaspoon garlic powder
⅛ teaspoon oregano

You'll need: medium bowl, skillet, nonstick spray

Prep: 5 minutes
Cook: 5 minutes

1. In a medium bowl, use a fork to whisk egg with seasonings.

2. Bring a skillet sprayed with nonstick spray to medium heat. Add spinach and tomato. Cook and stir until tomato is soft and spinach has wilted, 1 to 2 minutes.

3. Add seasoned egg. Scramble for 2 to 3 minutes, until fully cooked.

4. Stir in olives and feta, and cook and until hot, about 30 seconds.

MAKES 1 SERVING

SURVEY SAYS . . .

Wow! 69% of Hungry Girl fans prefer egg scrambles to sunny-side-up eggs.

DENVER OMELETTE BAKE

 ¼th of pan: 215 calories, 5.5g total fat (3g sat fat), 751mg sodium, 10g carbs, 1.5g fiber, 4g sugars, 29.5g protein

5

1 cup chopped **onion**
1 cup chopped **bell pepper**
2½ cups (about 20 large) **egg whites** or **fat-free liquid egg substitute**
6 ounces (about 9 slices) **reduced-sodium ham**, chopped
¾ cup shredded **reduced-fat cheddar cheese**

seasonings:
½ teaspoon onion powder
¼ teaspoon black pepper

You'll need: large oven-safe skillet, nonstick spray

Prep: 10 minutes
Cook: 55 minutes
Cool: 5 minutes

1. Preheat oven to 375 degrees.

2. Spray a large oven-safe skillet with nonstick spray, and bring to medium-high heat on the stove. Add onion and bell pepper, and cook and stir until slightly softened, about 4 minutes.

3. Remove skillet from heat, and let cool for 5 minutes.

4. Add egg, chopped ham, ½ cup cheddar, and seasonings. Gently mix.

5. Bake until center is firm, about 45 minutes.

6. Sprinkle with remaining ¼ cup cheddar. Bake until melted, about 5 minutes.

MAKES 4 SERVINGS

EXTRA, EXTRA!

Top with chopped chives. Fancy!

HG TIP!

If you're not sure if the skillet handle is oven safe, wrap it in aluminum foil first.

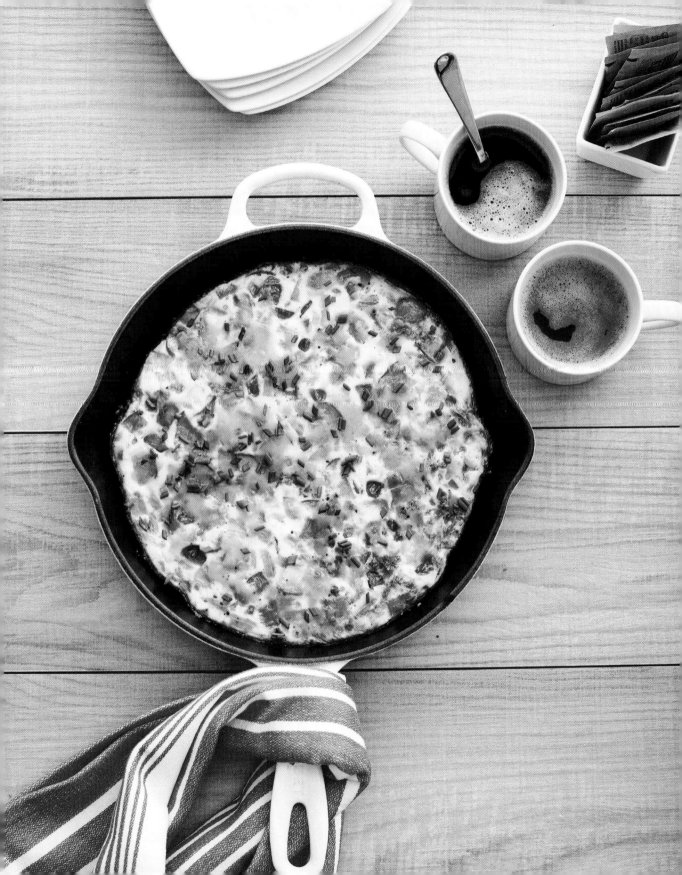

EASY FREEZY BREAKFAST SANDWICHES

 ¼th of recipe (1 sandwich): 214 calories, 4g total fat (2g sat fat), 600mg sodium, 27.5g carbs, 6.5g fiber, 2g sugars, 21.5g protein

4

1½ cups (about 12 large) **egg whites** or **fat-free liquid egg substitute**
4 **light English muffins**
4 slices (about 3 ounces) **reduced-sodium ham**
½ cup shredded **reduced-fat cheddar cheese**

seasonings:
½ teaspoon onion powder
⅛ teaspoon black pepper

You'll need: 8-inch by 8-inch baking pan, nonstick spray, medium-large bowl

Prep: 5 minutes
Cook: 25 minutes

1. Preheat oven to 375 degrees. Spray an 8-inch by 8-inch baking pan with nonstick spray.

2. In a medium-large bowl, use a fork to whisk egg with seasonings.

3. Transfer to the baking pan. Bake until firm and cooked through, 18 to 20 minutes.

4. Meanwhile, split and toast English muffins. Warm ham in the microwave, if desired.

5. Sprinkle cheese over the egg bake. Bake until melted, about 2 minutes.

6. Slice egg bake into 4 squares. If eating immediately, lay a square on top of each bottom muffin half. Top with ham. Finish with top muffin halves.

MAKES 4 SERVINGS

HG FYI

If you plan to eat these the same week they're made, no need to freeze! Just wrap in parchment paper and refrigerate.

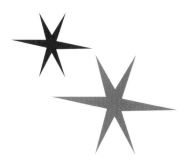

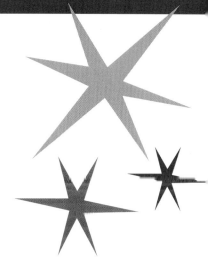

Freezing and Reheating

TO FREEZE

Before assembling sandwiches, let egg bake squares cool completely, about 30 minutes. Once assembled, tightly wrap each sandwich in plastic wrap or aluminum foil, and place them in a large sealable freezer bag (or container). Remove as much air as possible, and freeze for up to a month.

TO REHEAT

Unwrap one frozen sandwich, tightly wrap in a paper towel, and place on a microwave-safe plate. Microwave at 50 percent power for 1½ minutes. Microwave at full power for another 1½ minutes, or until cheese has melted and sandwich is hot.

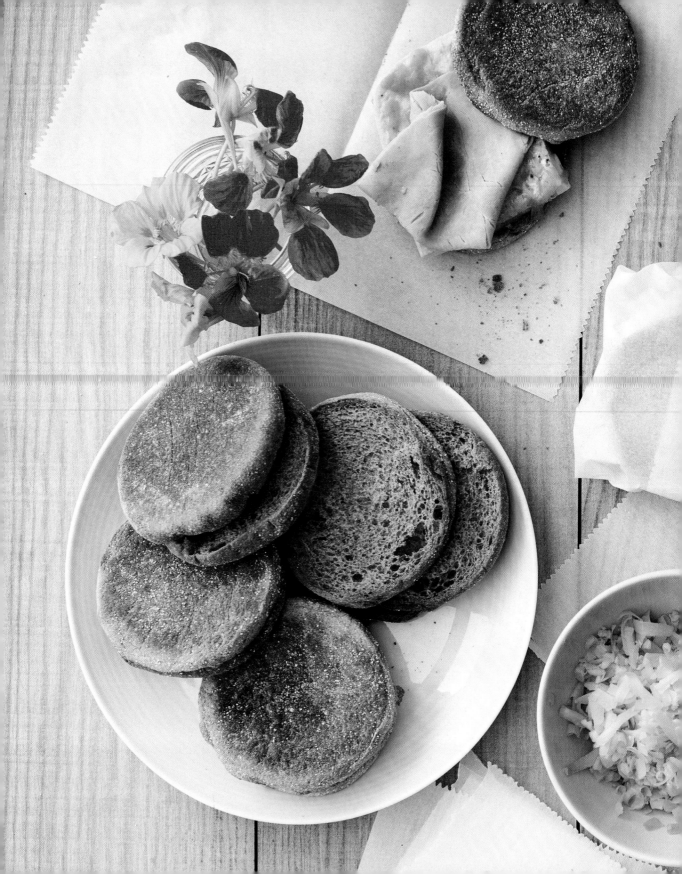

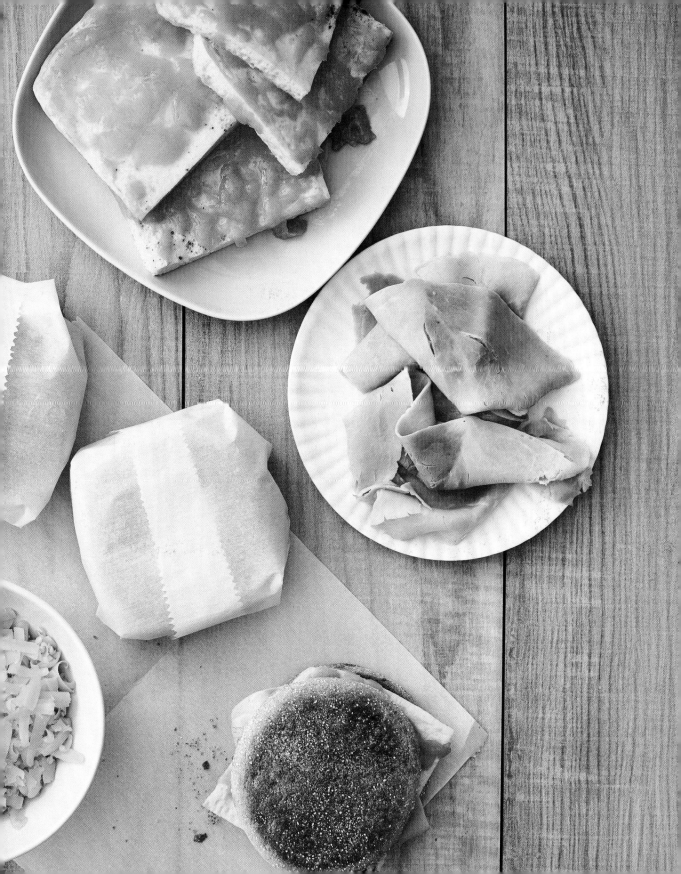

BROC 'N CHEDDAR CRUSTLESS QUICHE

V **GF** **¼th of pan:** 143 calories, 4.5g total fat (2.5g sat fat), 489mg sodium, 6g carbs, 1g fiber, 2.5g sugars, 18.5g protein

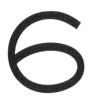

1½ cups roughly chopped **broccoli**
1½ cups (about 12 large) **egg whites** or **fat-free liquid egg substitute**
⅓ cup **fat-free plain Greek yogurt**
¼ cup **fat-free milk**
¾ cup shredded **reduced-fat cheddar cheese**
2 tablespoons chopped **scallions**

seasonings:
¼ teaspoon onion powder
¼ teaspoon garlic powder
¼ teaspoon each salt and black pepper

143 CALORIES

You'll need: 9-inch pie pan, nonstick spray, medium-large microwave-safe bowl, large bowl

Prep: 10 minutes
Cook: 30 minutes

1. Preheat oven to 375 degrees. Spray a 9-inch pie pan with nonstick spray.

2. Place broccoli in a medium-large microwave-safe bowl. Add ¼ cup water. Cover and microwave for 2½ minutes, or until soft. Drain excess liquid.

3. In a large bowl, combine egg, yogurt, milk, and seasonings. Whisk with a fork until uniform. Add broccoli and cheese, and stir to mix.

4. Transfer to the pie pan. Bake until firm and cooked through, about 25 minutes.

5. Top with scallions.

MAKES 4 SERVINGS

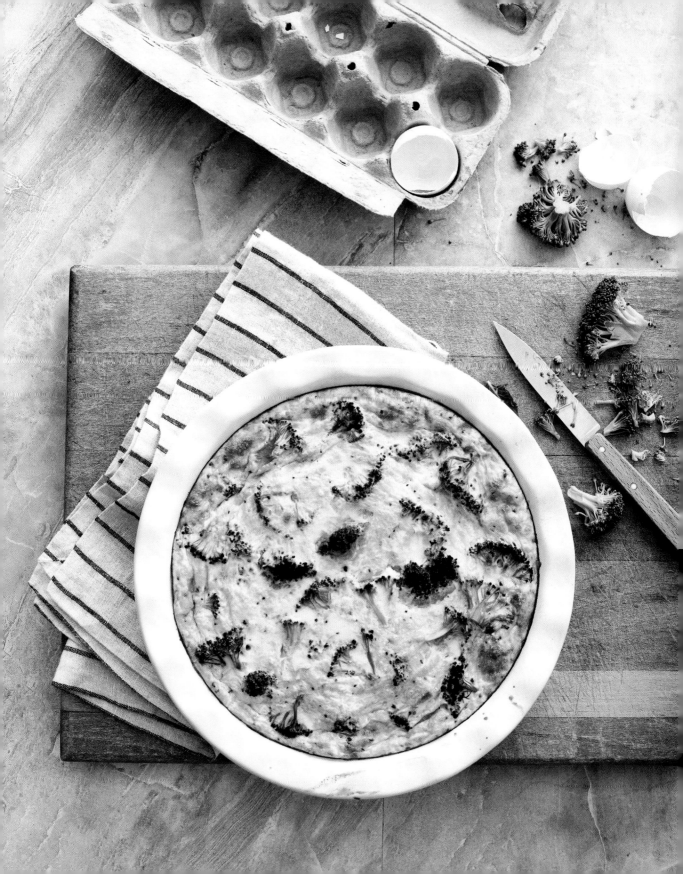

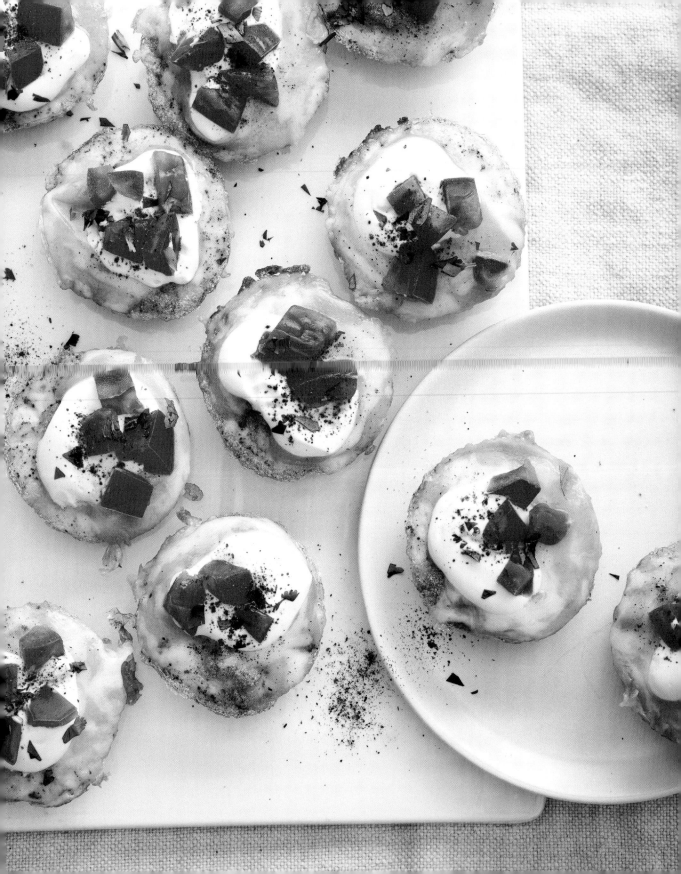

SOUTHWEST MUFFIN-PAN EGG BAKES

V GF **⅙th of recipe (2 egg bakes):** 142 calories, 4g total fat (2g sat fat), 388mg sodium, 9g carbs, 1.5g fiber, 2.5g sugars, 16.5g protein

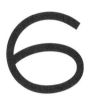

2½ cups (about 20 large) **egg whites** or **fat-free liquid egg substitute**
½ cup **canned black beans**, drained and rinsed
½ cup **frozen sweet corn kernels**
¾ cup shredded **reduced-fat Mexican-blend cheese**
¼ cup **light sour cream**
½ cup chopped **tomatoes**

seasonings:
1½ teaspoons taco seasoning, or more for topping

142 CALORIES

You'll need: 12-cup muffin pan, foil baking cups (or nonstick spray), large bowl

Prep: 15 minutes
Cook: 25 minutes

HG FYI

There's a recipe for DIY taco seasoning on page 358!

1 Preheat oven to 375 degrees. Line a 12-cup muffin pan with foil baking cups, or spray it with nonstick spray.

2. In a large bowl, use a fork to whisk egg with taco seasoning. Stir in beans and corn.

3. Evenly fill muffin pan. Bake until firm and cooked through, about 20 minutes.

4. Sprinkle with cheese. Bake until melted, about 3 minutes.

5. Top with sour cream and tomatoes.

MAKES 6 SERVINGS

EXTRA, EXTRA!

Sprinkle some cilantro on top for bonus flavor.

MUFFIN-PAN EGGS BENE-CHICK

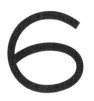

30m **GF** **¼th of recipe (3 egg cups):** 153 calories, 3.5g total fat (1.5g sat fat), 760mg sodium, 4.5g carbs, 0g fiber, 2g sugars, 22g protein

6

12 slices (about 8 ounces) **reduced-sodium ham**
1¾ cups (about 14 large) **egg whites** or **fat-free liquid egg substitute**
¼ cup **fat-free plain Greek yogurt**
1½ tablespoons **Dijon mustard**
1½ tablespoons **whipped butter**
¼ teaspoon **lemon juice**

seasonings:
½ teaspoon garlic powder
½ teaspoon onion powder

153 CALORIES

You'll need: 12-cup muffin pan, nonstick spray, large bowl, small microwave-safe bowl

Prep: 10 minutes
Cook: 15 minutes

1. Preheat oven to 400 degrees. Spray a 12-cup muffin pan with nonstick spray.

2. Press a ham slice into each cup of the muffin pan.

3. In a large bowl, use a fork to whisk egg with seasonings.

4. Evenly fill muffin pan. Bake until firm and cooked through, about 15 minutes.

5. Meanwhile, to make the sauce, mix remaining ingredients in a small microwave-safe bowl. Microwave for 30 seconds, or until hot.

6. Serve eggs topped with sauce.

MAKES 4 SERVINGS

EXTRA, EXTRA!

Top with salt and black pepper to taste.
Freshly cracked is the best!

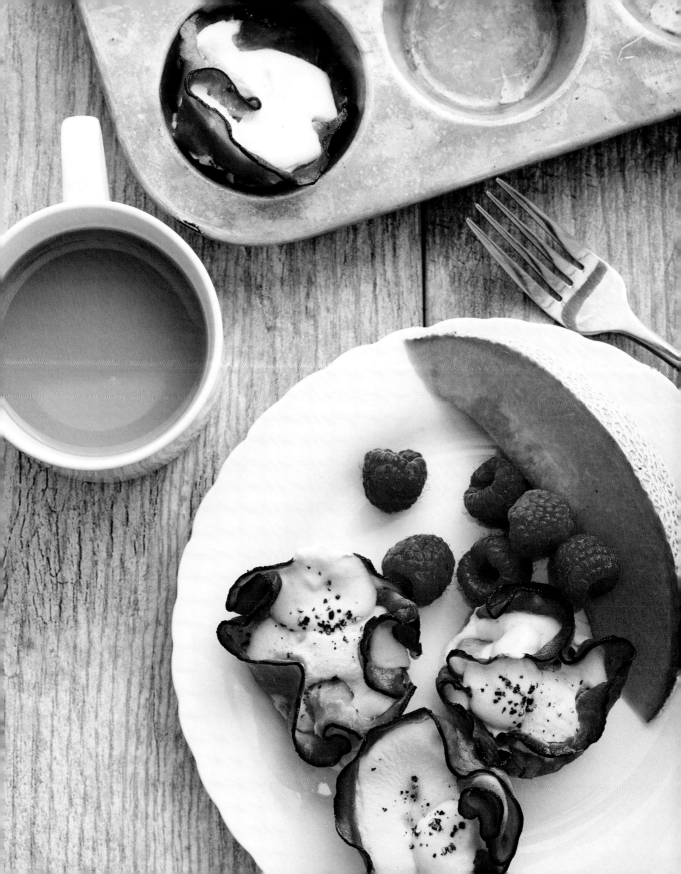

CLASSIC HARD-BOILED EGGS

30m **V** **GF** **¹⁄₁₂th of recipe (1 egg):** 72 calories, 4.5g total fat (1.5g sat fat), 71mg sodium, 0.5g carbs, 0g fiber, <0.5g sugars, 6g protein

1 | 12 **large eggs**

You'll need:
large pot

Prep: 5 minutes
Cook: 20 minutes

1. Place eggs in a pot, and cover with water, leaving a few inches of the pot's inner edge above the water line. Bring to a boil.

2. Once boiling, cook for 10 minutes.

MAKES 12 SERVINGS

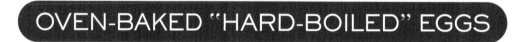

OVEN-BAKED "HARD-BOILED" EGGS

V **GF** **¹⁄₁₂th of recipe (1 egg):** 72 calories, 4.5g total fat (1.5g sat fat), 71mg sodium, 0.5g carbs, 0g fiber, <0.5g sugars, 6g protein

1 | 12 **large eggs**

You'll need: 12-cup muffin pan

Prep: 5 minutes
Cook: 30 minutes

1. Preheat oven to 350 degrees.

2. Place an egg (still in its shell) in each cup of the muffin pan.

3. Bake for 30 minutes.

MAKES 12 SERVINGS

HG FYI:

The shells may develop a few brown spots, but don't be concerned! The eggs inside will be A-OK.

INSTANT-POT HARD-BOILED EGGS

30m **V** **GF** **¹⁄₁₂th of recipe (1 egg):** 72 calories, 4.5g total fat (1.5g sat fat), 71mg sodium, 0.5g carbs, 0g fiber, <0.5g sugars, 6g protein

1 | 12 **large eggs**

72 CALORIES

You'll need:
Instant Pot

Prep: 5 minutes
Cook: 25 minutes

1. Add ¾ cup water to an Instant Pot. Place a stainless-steel steamer basket inside the pot.

2. Add eggs, and seal with lid. Press Manual, and set for 7 minutes.

3. Once cooked, press Keep Warm/Cancel to release steam.

MAKES 12 SERVINGS

HG FYI

Don't miss the Instant Pot primer on page 361!

ANOTHER HG FYI

Peeling these eggs is as easy as 1-2-3 . . .
Just flip to page 60!

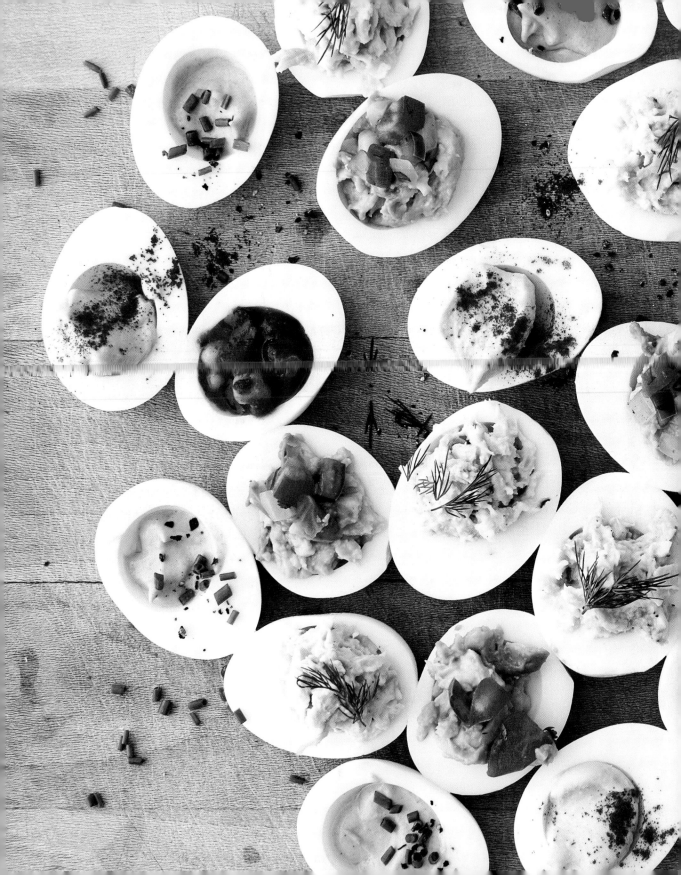

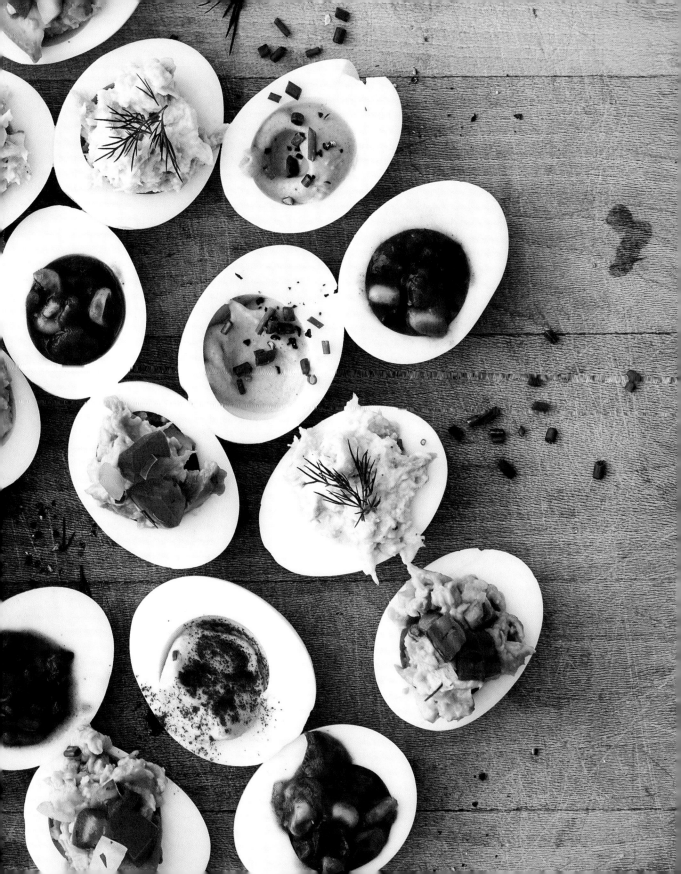

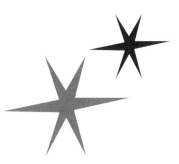

Peeling Hard-Boiled Eggs

Easy as 1-2-3!

STEP 1
Place eggs in a bowl, and cover with ice and cold water.

STEP 2
Let sit for 20 minutes.

STEP 3
Gently crack eggs on the rim of the bowl, and easily peel off the shells!

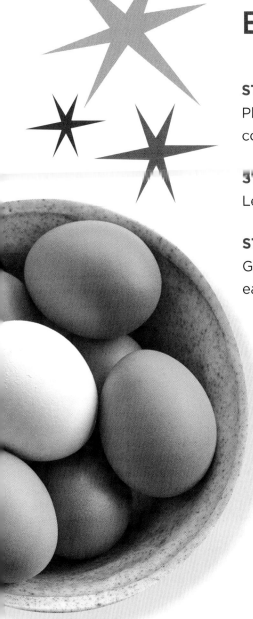

6 Snack Ideas for Hard-Boiled Eggs

Whether you cook 'em on the stove, in the oven, or in an Instant Pot, hard-boiled eggs ROCK. And while there's nothing wrong with the occasional yolk, I like to pop 'em out to make room for tasty fillings like these . . .

1. Salsa. Add zesty flavor with your favorite jarred salsa. My favorites are pineapple and black bean & corn salsa!

2. Hummus. Sorry, pita chips! Hummus has a new BFF. Fill your egg whites with this Mediterranean dip for a next-level snack.

3. Avocado. Mash it, season it, and top your egg whites with it. Yum!

4. Tuna. Pump up the protein! Whip up a DIY tuna salad with light mayo and seasonings . . . or reach for a pouch of the ready-to-eat stuff!

5. Bean Dip. Hummus isn't the only game in town. Bean dips are made with edamame, white beans, black beans, and more. Fill 'er up!

6. Dijon Mustard. Mix it with light mayo to mellow out the intensity. Mash in a yolk for a deviled egg fix!

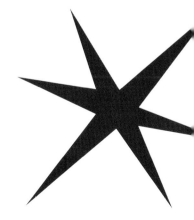

BAGELED EGGS

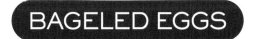

 ½ of recipe (6 egg white halves): 168 calories, 8.5g total fat (3.5g sat fat), 583mg sodium, 4g carbs, 0.5g fiber, 2g sugars, 17.5g protein

5

6 hard-boiled and chilled **large eggs**
2 tablespoons **light/reduced-fat cream cheese**
2 tablespoons finely chopped **red onion**
1 ounce **smoked salmon**, cut into 12 pieces
3 **cherry or grape tomatoes**, quartered

seasonings:
½ teaspoon everything bagel seasoning, or more for topping

You'll need: medium bowl

Prep: 10 minutes

1. Halve eggs lengthwise. Discard four yolks (or save for another use).

2. Place remaining two yolks in a medium bowl. Add cream cheese, onion, and seasoning. Mix until uniform.

3. Distribute salmon among egg white halves, followed by cream cheese mixture.

4. Top with quartered tomatoes.

MAKES 2 SERVINGS

HG FYIs

You can find ready-to-eat hard-boiled eggs in both the fridge and freezer sections at some supermarkets!

Everything bagel seasoning is ALWAYS in my spice drawer . . . I LOVE the kind by Trader Joe's! There's also a DIY recipe on page 357.

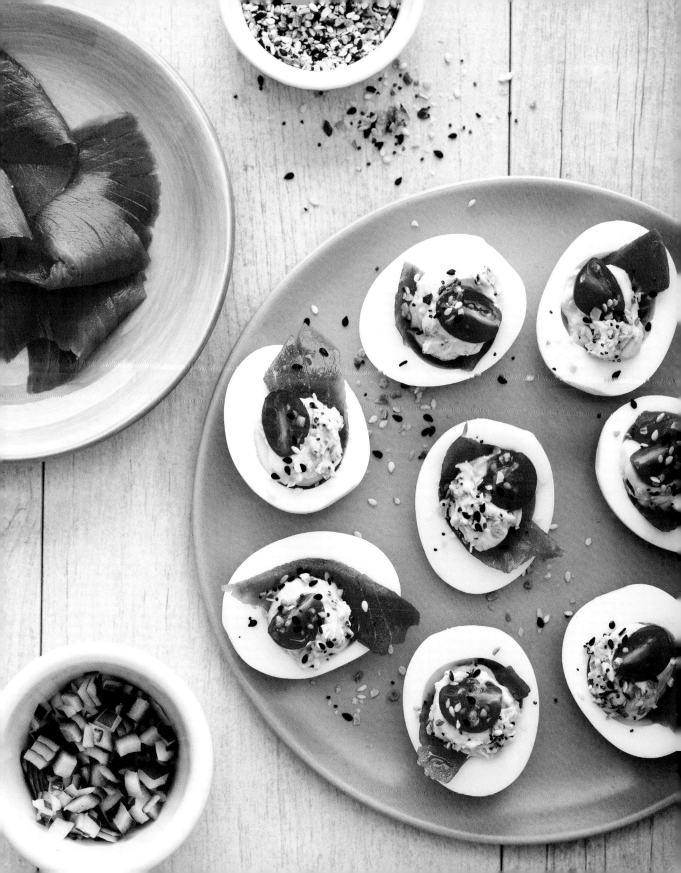

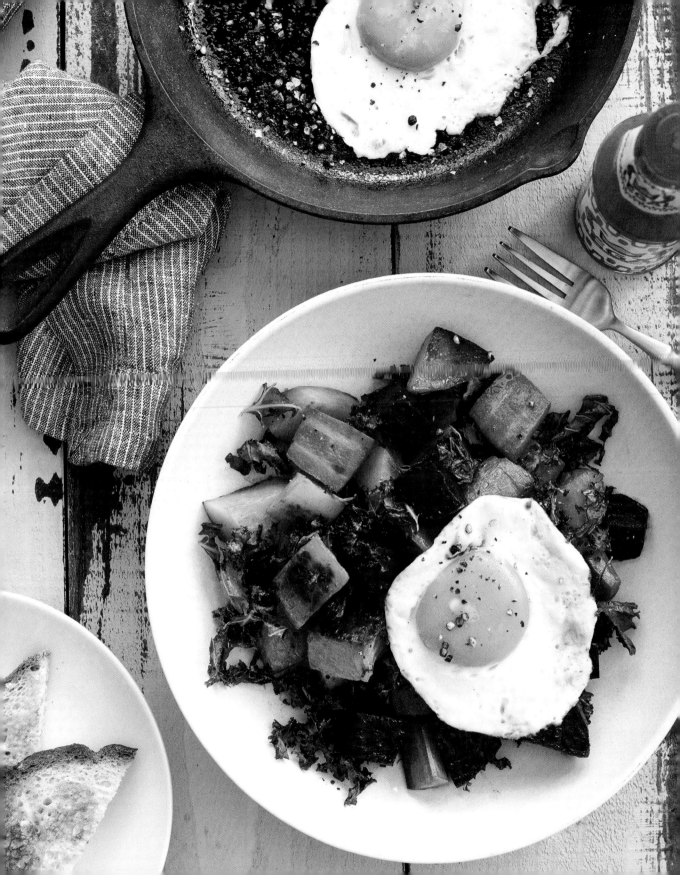

ROASTED VEGGIE EGG POWER BOWL

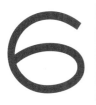 **Entire recipe:** 288 calories, 12.5g total fat (2.5g sat fat), 657mg sodium, 37g carbs, 9g fiber, 13.5g sugars, 11.5g protein

6

1 cup (about ¼th of a medium) peeled **butternut squash** cut into 1-inch chunks
¾ cup (about 1 large) peeled **carrot** cut into 1-inch chunks
½ cup (about 1) peeled **beet** cut into 1-inch chunks
1½ teaspoons **olive oil**
2 cups chopped **kale**
1 **large egg**

seasonings:
⅛ teaspoon plus a dash each salt and black pepper
⅛ teaspoon garlic powder
⅛ teaspoon onion powder

288 CALORIES

You'll need: baking sheet, nonstick spray, large bowl, medium bowl, skillet

Prep: 10 minutes
Cook: 30 minutes

1. Preheat oven to 400 degrees. Spray a baking sheet with nonstick spray.

2. In a large bowl, combine squash, carrot, beet, 1 teaspoon oil, and ⅛ teaspoon of each seasoning. Toss to coat.

3. Evenly distribute onto half of the baking sheet. Bake for 18 minutes.

4. Meanwhile, in the large bowl, mix kale with remaining ½ teaspoon oil and dash each salt and pepper.

5. Flip veggies on baking sheet, and add kale to the other half. Bake until kale is slightly crispy and other veggies are softened and browned, about 10 minutes.

6. Transfer veggies to a medium bowl.

7. Bring a skillet sprayed with nonstick spray to medium heat. Cook egg sunny-side up, 1 to 2 minutes. (Or cook to your preference.)

8. Place egg over veggies.

MAKES 1 SERVING

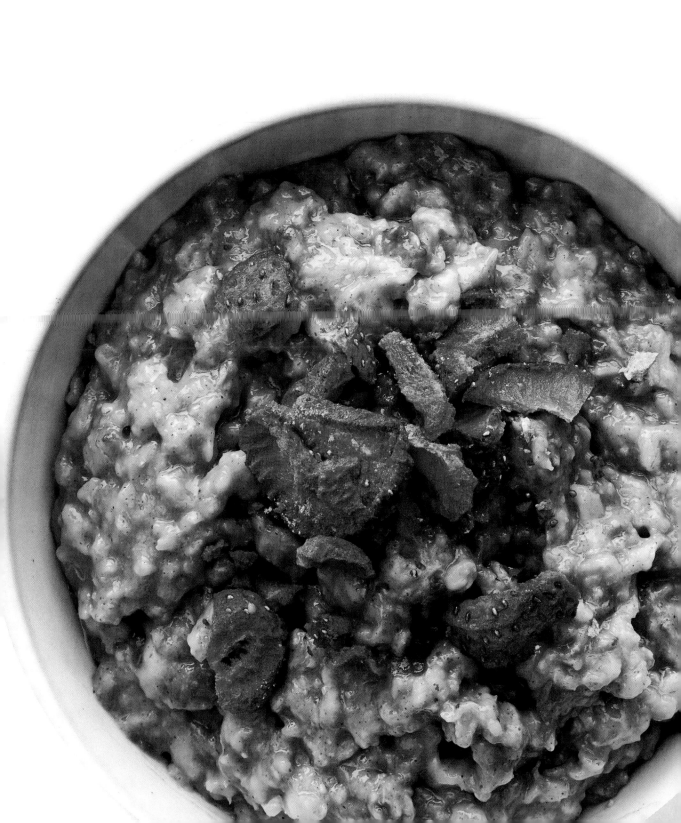

2

SIMPLY OATS

Muffins, pancakes, breakfast cookies & more. Plus, the simplest oatmeal recipes ever and the baking appliance you never knew you needed. (Hint: It's usually reserved for smoothies.)

SIMPLE GROWING OATMEAL

V **GF** **Entire recipe:** 194 calories, 5.5g fat (0.5g sat fat), 333mg sodium, 30g carbs, 5g fiber, 1.5g sugars, 6.5g protein

1 cup **unsweetened vanilla almond milk**
½ cup **old-fashioned oats**
¼ teaspoon **vanilla extract**
1 packet **natural no-calorie sweetener**

seasonings:
⅛ teaspoon cinnamon
Dash salt

194 CALORIES

You'll need:
nonstick pot, medium bowl

Prep: 5 minutes
Cook: 20 minutes
Cool: 10 minutes

1. In a nonstick pot, combine milk, oats, extract, and seasonings.

2. Stir in 1 cup water, and bring to a boil.

3. Reduce to a simmer. Cook and stir until thick and creamy, 12 to 15 minutes.

4. Transfer to a medium bowl, and stir in sweetener. Let cool until thickened, 5 to 10 minutes.

MAKES 1 SERVING

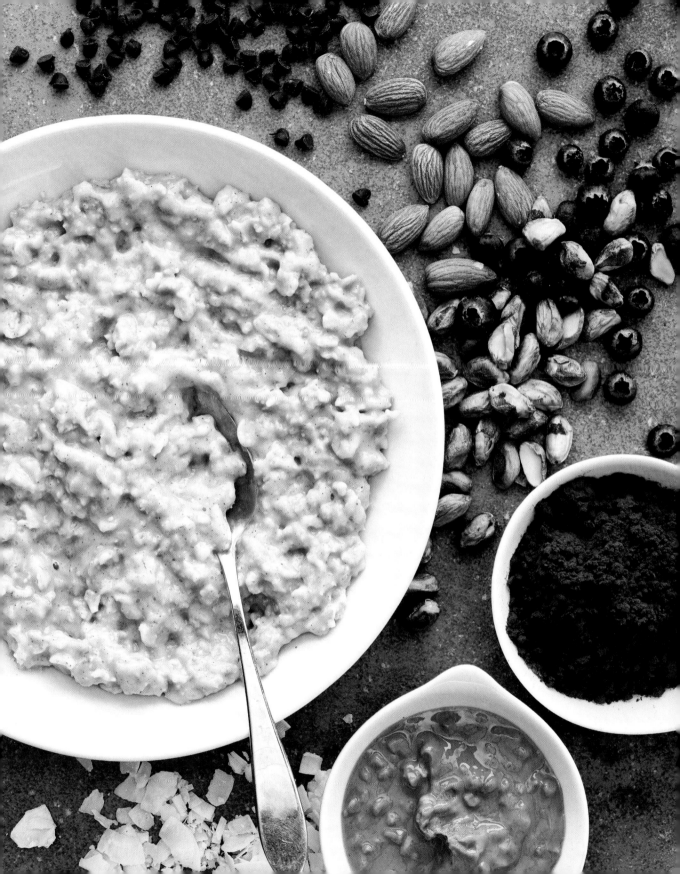

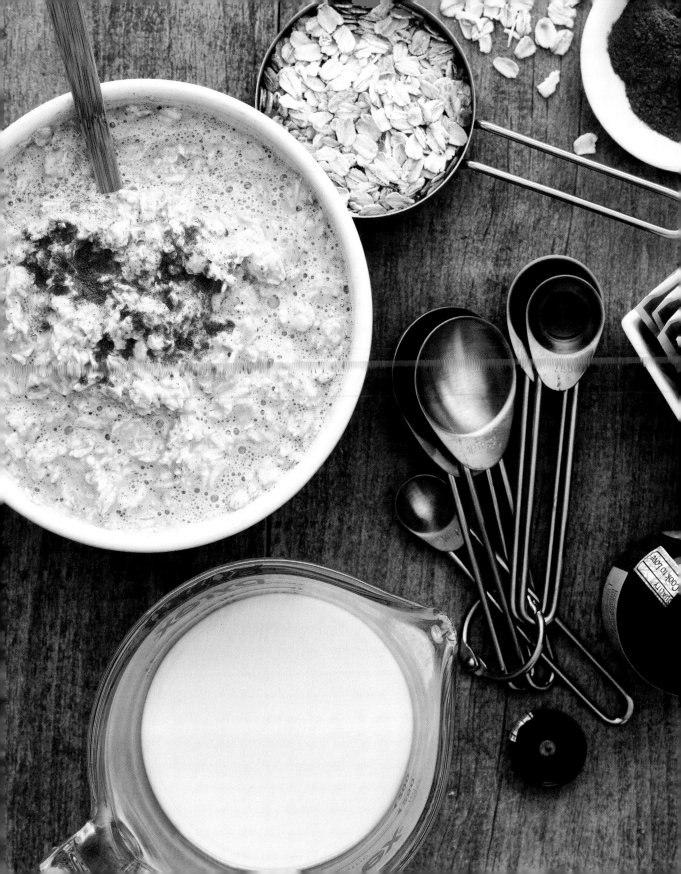

SIMPLE OVERNIGHT OATS

 Entire recipe: 177 calories, 4g total fat (0.5g sat fat), 244mg sodium, 29g carbs, 4.5g fiber, 1g sugars, 6g protein

4

½ cup **old-fashioned oats**
½ cup **unsweetened vanilla almond milk**
¼ teaspoon **vanilla extract**
1 packet **natural no-calorie sweetener**

seasonings:
Dash cinnamon, or more for topping
Dash salt

You'll need: medium bowl or jar

Prep: 5 minutes
Chill: 6 hours

1. In a medium bowl or jar, combine all ingredients and seasonings. Mix well.

2. Cover and refrigerate for at least 6 hours, until oats are soft and have absorbed most of the liquid.

MAKES 1 SERVING

6 Ways to Dress Up Oatmeal

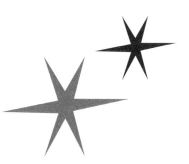

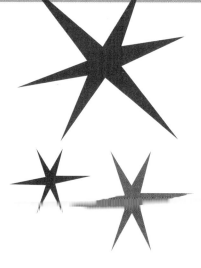

Rock the Oat

My Simple Growing Oatmeal and Simple Overnight Oats recipes are the perfect bases for personalized oatmeal bowls. Check out these toppings and add-in ideas . . . Then mix & match!

1. Fruit. Whether fresh, thawed from frozen, or freeze-dried, fruit adds sweetness, texture, and volume to oatmeal. I can't think of a single fruit that WOULDN'T taste great with oats.

2. Greek Yogurt. Make a parfait by layering fat-free Greek yogurt with chilled oatmeal, or just add a dollop on top! Keep it classic with vanilla or experiment with lots of flavors.

3. Nuts. Crunch + healthy fats = no brainer! My top picks are sliced almonds, pistachios, and chopped peanuts. A little goes a long way . . .

4. Powdered Peanut Butter. Stir in a spoonful of powdered peanut butter to add major flavor without a lot of calories. Or mix it with water and drizzle over your oats!

5. Chocolate. Mini semi-sweet chocolate chips and/or unsweetened cocoa powder will make your breakfast taste like dessert. Dark cocoa adds extra richness!

6. Extracts. Vanilla isn't your only option. Try almond, coconut, rum, hazelnut, and more . . . Have fun and experiment!

Steel Cut vs. Old Fashioned

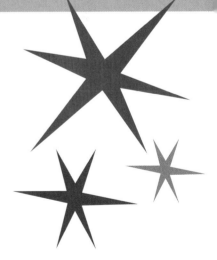

Vote for Oats

Curious about the differences between these two types of oats? Steel-cut oats are coarsely chopped, which produces a heartier, chewier oatmeal. Old-fashioned oats have been steamed, rolled flat, and toasted . . . Oatmeal made with these oats has a softer, porridge-like consistency. I've got recipes featuring each kind. Find your new favorite!

BLUEBERRY PIE GROWING OATMEAL

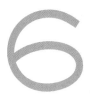

V **GF** **Entire recipe:** 237 calories, 5.5g total fat (0.5g sat fat), 487mg sodium, 40.5g carbs, 6g fiber, 6g sugars, 6.5g protein

6

1 cup **unsweetened vanilla almond milk**
½ cup **old-fashioned oats**
¼ teaspoon **vanilla extract**
2 packets **natural no-calorie sweetener**
1 teaspoon **cornstarch**
⅓ cup **blueberries** (fresh or thawed from frozen and drained; no sugar added)

seasonings:
⅛ teaspoon plus a dash cinnamon
2 dashes salt

237 CALORIES

You'll need:
nonstick pot, two medium bowls (one microwave-safe)

Prep: 5 minutes
Cook: 20 minutes
Cool: 10 minutes

1. In a nonstick pot, combine milk, oats, vanilla extract, ⅛ teaspoon cinnamon, and a dash of salt.

2. Stir in 1 cup water, and bring to a boil.

3. Reduce to a simmer. Cook and stir until thick and creamy, 12 to 15 minutes.

4. Transfer to a medium bowl, and stir in 1 sweetener packet. Let cool until thickened, 5 to 10 minutes.

5. Meanwhile, in a medium microwave-safe bowl, combine cornstarch with 2 teaspoons water. Stir to dissolve. Add blueberries and remaining sweetener packet, dash of cinnamon, and dash of salt. Mix well. Cover and microwave until hot and thickened, about 1 minute.

6. Mix well, and spoon over oatmeal.

MAKES 1 SERVING

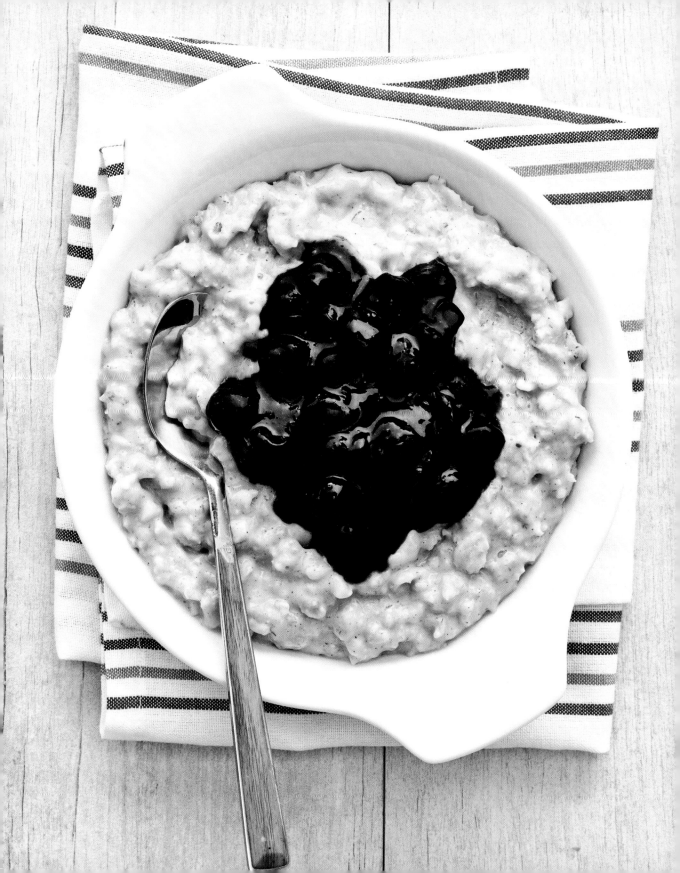

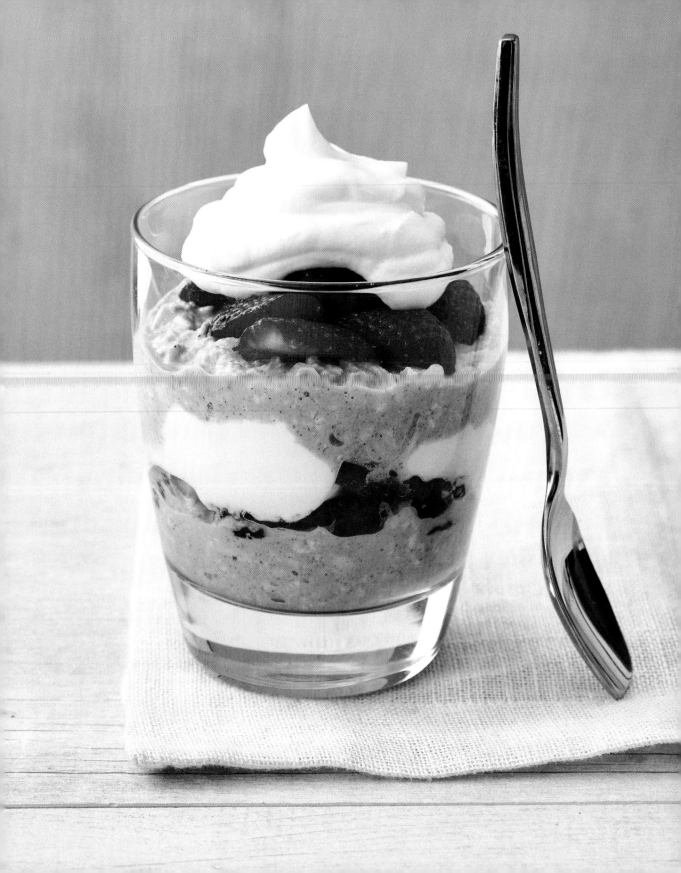

PB&J OVERNIGHT OAT PARFAIT

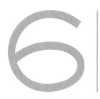 **Entire recipe:** 335 calories, 6g total fat (0.5g sat fat), 177mg sodium, 46.5g carbs, 7.5g fiber, 12g sugars, 26.5g protein

6

½ cup **old-fashioned oats**
½ cup **unsweetened vanilla almond milk**
1½ tablespoons **powdered peanut butter**
3 packets **natural no-calorie sweetener**
⅔ cup **fat-free plain Greek yogurt**
½ cup sliced **strawberries**

seasonings:
¼ teaspoon cinnamon

You'll need: medium bowl, small bowl, tall glass or jar

Prep: 5 minutes
Chill: 6 hours

1. In a medium bowl, combine oats, milk, powdered peanut butter, 1½ sweetener packets, and ⅛ teaspoon cinnamon. Add 2 tablespoons water, and mix well.

2. Cover and refrigerate for at least 6 hours, until oats are soft and have absorbed most of the liquid.

3. In a small bowl, mix Greek yogurt with remaining 1½ sweetener packets and ⅛ teaspoon cinnamon.

4. Stir oatmeal. In a tall glass or jar, layer half of each ingredient: oatmeal, strawberries, and yogurt. Repeat layering.

MAKES 1 SERVING

INSTANT-POT STRAWBERRY BANANA OATMEAL

V **GF** **¼th of recipe (about 1¼ cups):** 273 calories, 4.5g total fat (0.5g sat fat), 236mg sodium, 51.5g carbs, 8.5g fiber, 14.5g sugars, 6.5g protein

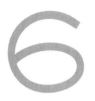

2 cups **unsweetened vanilla almond milk**
2 cups **old-fashioned oats**
1 cup (about 2 medium) mashed **extra-ripe bananas**
4 packets **natural no-calorie sweetener**
1 tablespoon **vanilla extract**
1½ cups chopped **freeze-dried strawberries**, or more for topping

seasonings:
2 teaspoons cinnamon
⅛ teaspoon salt

273 CALORIES

You'll need: Instant Pot, nonstick spray

Prep: 5 minutes
Cook: 25 minutes
Cool: 5 minutes

1. In an Instant Pot sprayed with nonstick spray, combine milk, oats, bananas, sweetener, vanilla extract, and seasonings. Add 1 cup freeze-dried strawberries and 1½ cups water. Mix well.

2. Seal with lid. Press Multigrain, and set for 6 minutes.

3. Once cooked, press Keep Warm/Cancel. Let sit for 5 minutes.

4. Vent to release steam. Gently stir before serving.

5. Top each serving with 2 tablespoons of the remaining freeze-dried strawberries.

MAKES 4 SERVINGS

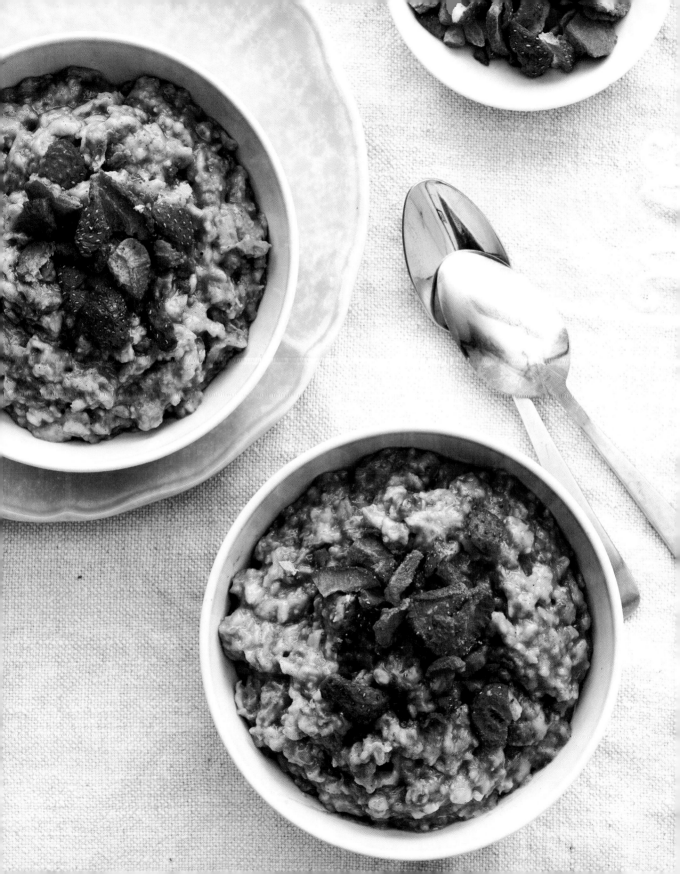

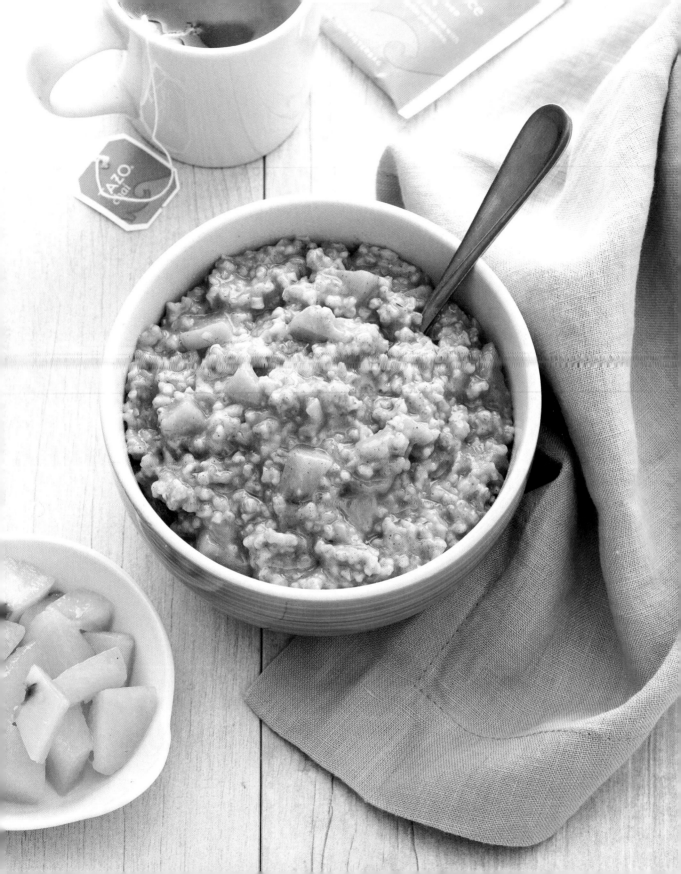

INSTANT-POT PEACHES 'N DREAM OATMEAL

 **¼th of recipe (1 heaping cup):** 223 calories, 4g total fat (0.5g sat fat), 235mg sodium, 38g carbs, 6.5g fiber, 7.5g sugars, 7g protein

5

2 cups chopped **peaches** (fresh or thawed from frozen; no sugar added)
2 cups **unsweetened vanilla almond milk**
1 cup **steel-cut oats**
5 packets **natural no-calorie sweetener**
1 tablespoon **vanilla extract**

seasonings:
2 teaspoons cinnamon
¼ teaspoon salt

223 CALORIES

You'll need: Instant Pot, nonstick spray

Prep: 10 minutes
Cook: 30 minutes
Cool: 10 minutes

1. Spray an Instant Pot with nonstick spray. Add ingredients, seasonings, and 1 cup water. Mix well.

2. Seal with lid. Press Manual, and set for 13 minutes.

3. Once cooked, press Keep Warm/Cancel. Let sit for 10 minutes.

4. Vent to release steam. Gently stir before serving.

MAKES 4 SERVINGS

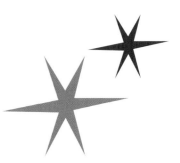

Batter in a Blender!

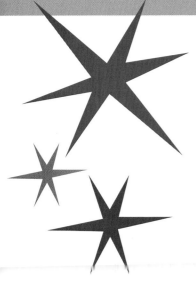

Your New Favorite Kitchen Hack

KITCHEN CLEANUP JUST GOT EASIER

Just like cooking eggs in a mug saves you from cleaning a skillet and spatula, making batter in a blender spares you the hassle of washing multiple mixing bowls and spoons. Forget separately stirring together the wet and dry ingredients for these recipes . . . Blender blades yield a perfectly uniform batter with the press of a button.

ANOTHER REASON I LOVE THE BLENDER-BATTER TECHNIQUE?

Oats are a wonderfully healthy ingredient, but the texture can be a bit coarse in pancakes and baked goods. The blender pulverizes those oats, so you get all the health benefits in the form of a flour!

For more blender batter favorites, check out the cookie recipes in the "Simply More . . . Sweets!" chapter, starting on page 327!

6 Simple Pancake Toppers

Top It Like It's Hot!

These pancakes are perfectly delicious on their own, but a little extra something never hurts . . .

1. Natural Sugar-Free Pancake Syrup

2. Whipped Butter

3. Powdered Sugar

4. Fresh Fruit

5. Fat-Free Greek Yogurt

6. Fruit Jam or Preserves

PB 'NANA BLENDER PANCAKES

30m **V** **GF** **½ of recipe (2 pancakes):** 235 calories, 6.5g total fat (1g sat fat), 454mg sodium, 31.5g carbs, 5.5g fiber, 8.5g sugars, 14.5g protein

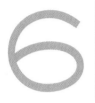

½ cup **old-fashioned oats**
½ cup (about 1 medium) mashed **extra-ripe banana**
½ cup (about 4 large) **egg whites** or **fat-free liquid egg substitute**
2 tablespoons **powdered peanut butter**
1 tablespoon **creamy peanut butter**
1 teaspoon **baking powder**

seasonings:
½ teaspoon cinnamon
Dash salt

235
CALORIES

You'll need: blender, skillet, nonstick spray

Prep: 5 minutes
Cook: 15 minutes

1. Add ingredients and seasonings to a blender, and blend until smooth.

2. Bring a skillet sprayed with nonstick spray to medium heat. Form a large pancake with ¼th of the batter, about ¼ cup. Cook until bubbles form and it's solid enough to flip, 1 to 2 minutes.

3. Gently flip, and cook until lightly browned and cooked through, about 1 minute.

4. Remove pancake. Remove skillet from heat, respray, and return to medium heat. Repeat to make 3 more pancakes.

MAKES 2 SERVINGS

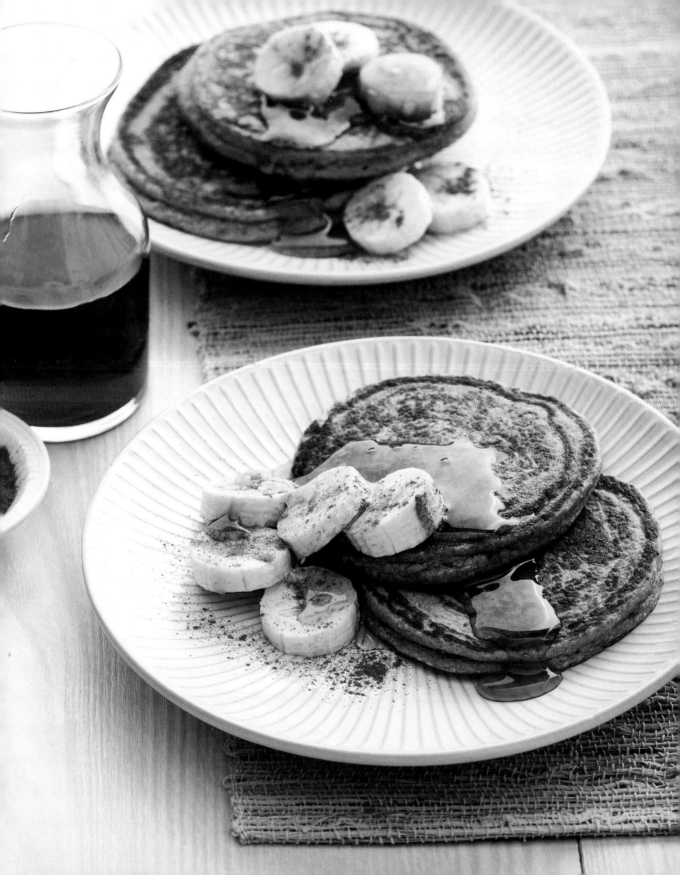

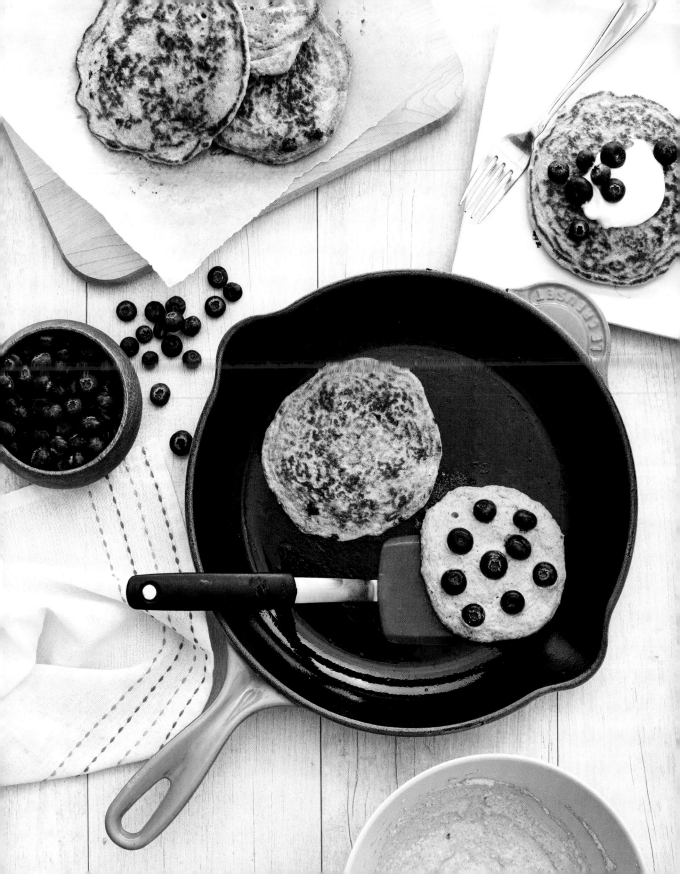

BLUEBERRY LEMON BLENDER PANCAKES

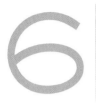 **½ of recipe (2 pancakes):** 194 calories, 2g total fat (<0.5g sat fat), 446mg sodium, 29.5g carbs, 3.5g fiber, 8.5g sugars, 15g protein

⅔ cup **old-fashioned oats**
½ cup **fat-free vanilla Greek yogurt**
½ cup (about 4 large) **egg whites** or **fat-free liquid egg substitute**
1 teaspoon **baking powder**
1 **lemon**
¼ cup **blueberries**

seasonings:
½ teaspoon cinnamon
Dash salt

You'll need: blender, fine grater or zester, skillet, nonstick spray

Prep: 5 minutes
Cook: 15 minutes

1. In a blender, combine oats, yogurt, egg, baking powder, and seasonings. Add 1 teaspoon lemon zest and 1½ teaspoons lemon juice.

2. Blend until smooth.

3. Bring a skillet sprayed with nonstick spray to medium heat. Form a large pancake with ¼th of the batter (about ¼ cup). Top with 1 tablespoon blueberries. Cook until bubbles form and it's solid enough to flip, 1 to 2 minutes.

4. Gently flip, and cook until lightly browned and cooked through, about 1 minute.

5. Remove pancake. Remove skillet from heat, respray, and return to medium heat. Repeat to make 3 more pancakes.

MAKES 2 SERVINGS

STRAWBERRY BANANA BLENDER PANCAKES

 30m **V** **GF** ½ **of recipe (2 pancakes):** 192 calories, 2g total fat (0.5g sat fat), 427mg sodium, 34g carbs, 5g fiber, 8.5g sugars, 10.5g protein

5

⅔ cup **old-fashioned oats**
½ cup (about 1 medium) mashed **extra-ripe banana**
½ cup (about 4 large) **egg whites** or **fat-free liquid egg substitute**
1 teaspoon **baking powder**
¼ cup chopped **strawberries**

seasonings:
½ teaspoon cinnamon
Dash salt

192
CALORIES

You'll need: blender, skillet, nonstick spray

Prep: 5 minutes
Cook: 10 minutes

1. In a blender, combine oats, banana, egg, baking powder, and seasonings.

2. Blend until smooth.

3. Bring a skillet sprayed with nonstick spray to medium heat. Form a large pancake with ¼th of the batter (about ¼ cup). Top with 1 tablespoon strawberries. Cook until bubbles form and it's solid enough to flip, 1 to 2 minutes.

4. Gently flip, and cook until lightly browned and cooked through, about 1 minute.

5. Remove pancake. Remove skillet from heat, respray, and return to medium heat. Repeat to make 3 more pancakes.

MAKES 2 SERVINGS

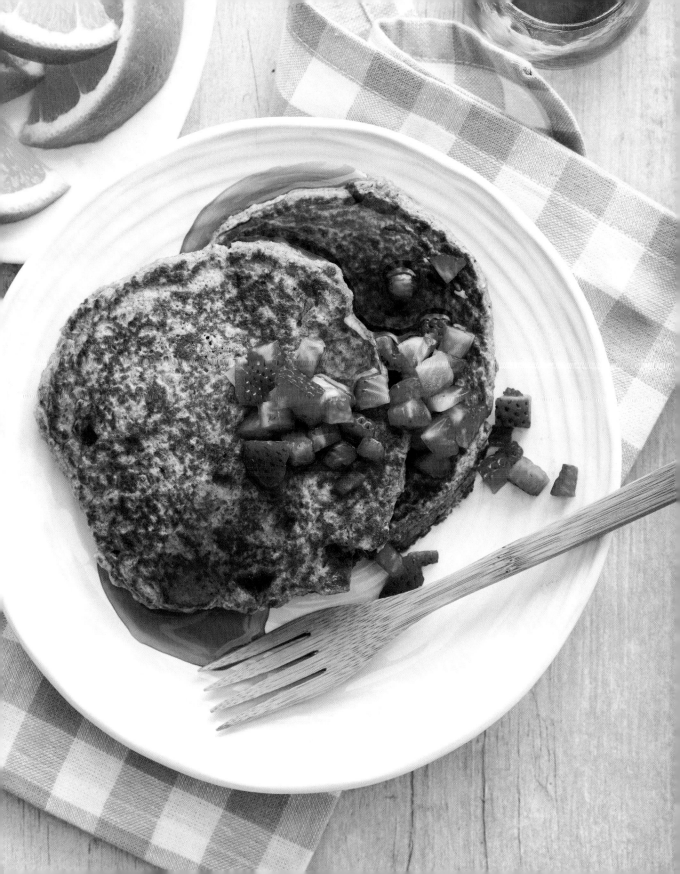

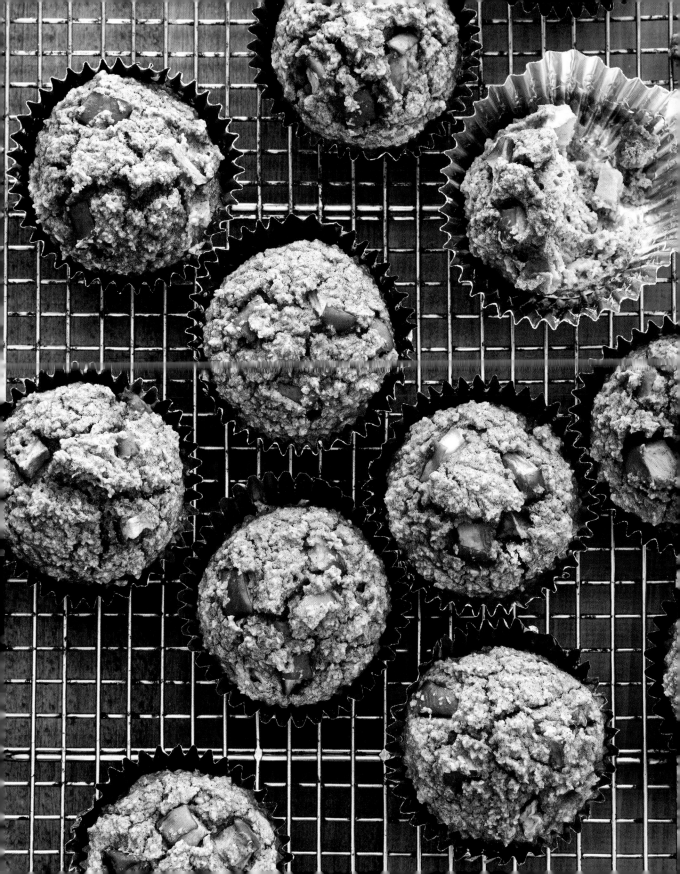

APPLE SPICE BLENDER MUFFINS

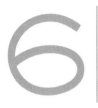 **30m** **V** **GF** **¹⁄₁₂th of recipe (1 muffin):** 93 calories, 1.5g total fat (<0.5g total fat), 168mg sodium, 16g carbs, 2.5g fiber, 1.5g sugars, 4g protein

3 cups **old-fashioned oats**
1½ cups **unsweetened vanilla almond milk**
½ cup (about 4 large) **egg whites** or **fat-free liquid egg substitute**
5 packets **natural no-calorie sweetener**
2 teaspoons **baking powder**
1 cup (about 1 medium) finely chopped **Fuji or Gala apple**

seasonings:
1 tablespoon pumpkin pie spice
¼ teaspoon salt

93 CALORIES

You'll need: 12-cup muffin pan, foil baking cups (or nonstick spray), blender

Prep: 10 minutes
Cook: 20 minutes

1. Preheat oven to 400 degrees. Line a 12-cup muffin pan with foil baking cups, or spray it with nonstick spray.

2. Place oats in a blender, and pulse to the consistency of coarse flour.

3. Add milk, egg, sweetener, baking powder, and seasonings. Blend until smooth and uniform, stopping and stirring if needed.

4. Stir apple into batter. Evenly fill muffin pan.

5. Bake until a knife inserted into the center of a muffin comes out clean, 16 to 18 minutes.

MAKES 12 SERVINGS

BLUEBERRY BLENDER MUFFINS

 ¹⁄₁₂th of recipe (1 muffin): 95 calories, 1.5g total fat (<0.5g sat fat), 168mg sodium, 16.5g carbs, 2.5g fiber, 2g sugars, 4g protein

6

3 cups **old-fashioned oats**
1½ cups **unsweetened vanilla almond milk**
½ cup (about 4 large) **egg whites** or **fat-free liquid egg substitute**
4 packets **natural no-calorie sweetener**
2 teaspoons **baking powder**
1 cup **blueberries** (fresh or thawed from frozen; no sugar added)

seasonings:
1½ teaspoons cinnamon
¼ teaspoon salt

You'll need: 12-cup muffin pan, foil baking cups (or nonstick spray), blender

Prep: 10 minutes
Cook: 20 minutes

1. Preheat oven to 400 degrees. Line a 12-cup muffin pan with foil baking cups, or spray it with nonstick spray.

2. In a blender, pulse oats to the consistency of coarse flour.

3. Add milk, egg, sweetener, baking powder, and seasonings. Blend until completely smooth and uniform, stopping and stirring if needed.

4. Stir blueberries into batter. Evenly fill muffin pan.

5. Bake until a knife inserted into the center of a muffin comes out clean, 16 to 18 minutes.

MAKES 12 SERVINGS

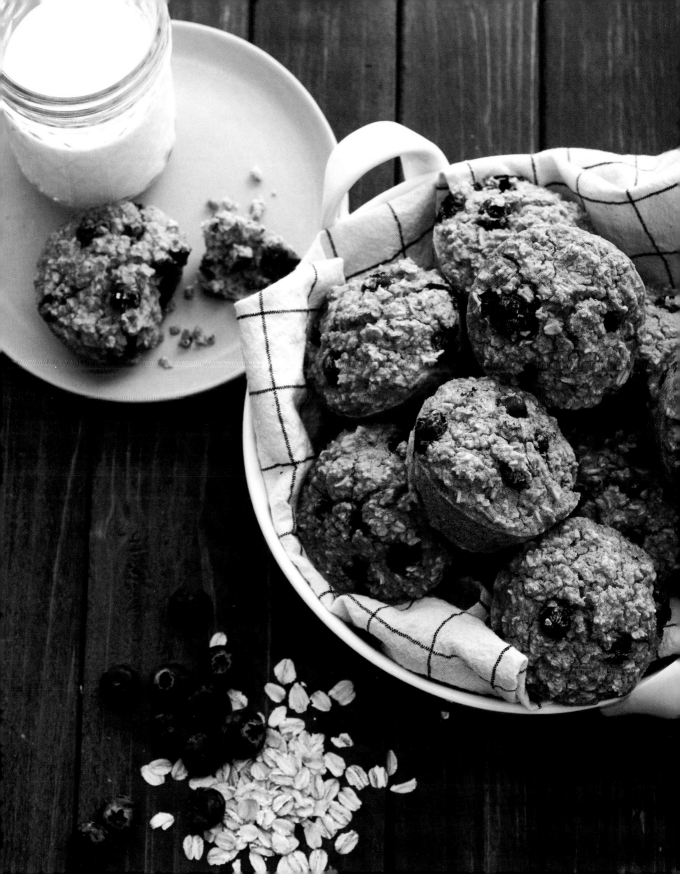

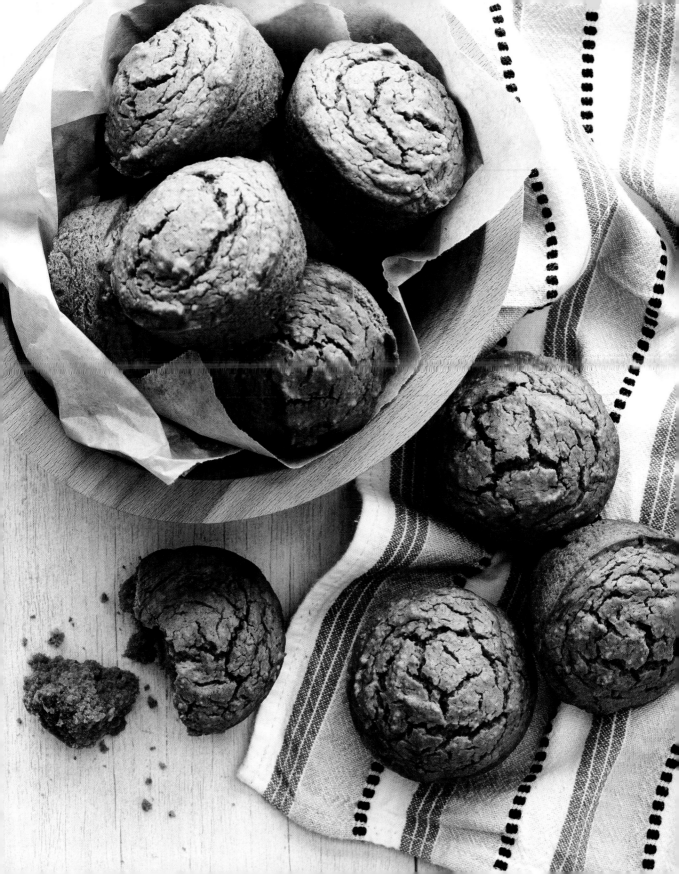

PB PROTEIN BLENDER MUFFINS

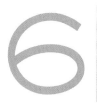 **1/12th of recipe (1 muffin):** 155 calories, 9g total fat (1g sat fat), 250mg sodium, 21g carbs, 3g fiber, 1.5g sugars, 9.5g protein

6

1 cup **old-fashioned oats**
1 cup **powdered peanut butter**
⅔ cup **Truvia spoonable no-calorie sweetener**
⅔ cup **creamy peanut butter**
⅔ cup (about 4 large) **egg whites** or **fat-free liquid egg substitute**
1¼ teaspoons **baking soda**

seasonings:
½ teaspoon cinnamon
¼ teaspoon salt

155 CALORIES

You'll need: 12-cup muffin pan, foil baking cups (or nonstick spray), blender

Prep: 10 minutes
Cook: 20 minutes

1. Preheat oven to 350 degrees. Line a 12-cup muffin pan with foil baking cups, or spray them with nonstick spray.

2. Place oats in a blender, and pulse to the consistency of coarse flour.

3. Add remaining ingredients, seasonings, and ¾ cup water. Blend until smooth and uniform, stopping and stirring if needed. (Batter will be thick.)

4. Evenly fill muffin pan, and smooth out the tops.

5. Bake until a knife inserted into the center of a muffin comes out clean, 16 to 18 minutes.

MAKES 12 SERVINGS

CINNAMON RAISIN BLENDER BREAKFAST COOKIES

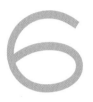 **30m** **V** **GF** **⅙th of recipe (1 cookie):** 158 calories, 2g total fat (0.5g sat fat), 216mg sodium, 27g carbs, 3.5g fiber, 7g sugars, 8.5g protein

2 cups **old-fashioned oats**
½ cup **unsweetened applesauce**
½ cup (about 4 large) **egg whites** or **fat-free liquid egg substitute**
⅓ cup (about 1 standard scoop) **vanilla protein powder**
1½ teaspoons **baking powder**
¼ cup **raisins**, chopped

seasonings:
2 teaspoons cinnamon
⅛ teaspoon salt

158 CALORIES

You'll need: baking sheet, parchment paper, blender

Prep: 10 minutes
Cook: 15 minutes

1. Preheat oven to 350 degrees. Line a baking sheet with parchment paper.

2. In a blender, pulse 1½ cups oats to the consistency of coarse flour.

3. Add applesauce, egg, protein powder, baking powder, seasonings, and ¼ cup water. Blend until smooth and uniform, stopping and stirring if needed.

4. Stir in remaining ½ cup oats and 2 tablespoons chopped raisins.

5. Evenly distribute batter into 6 mounds on the baking sheet, about ⅓ cup each. With the back of a spoon, lightly flatten into 5-inch circles.

6. Sprinkle with remaining 2 tablespoons chopped raisins, and lightly press to adhere. Bake until a knife inserted into the center of a cookie comes out clean, 10 to 12 minutes.

MAKES 6 SERVINGS

Protein Powder 411!

Look for protein powder that has about 100 calories per serving, usually about 1 ounce or 1 full scoop. That serving is equal to about ⅓ cup. Check out the smoothies in Chapter 8 for more protein powder magic!

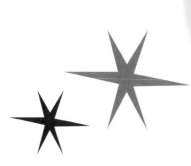

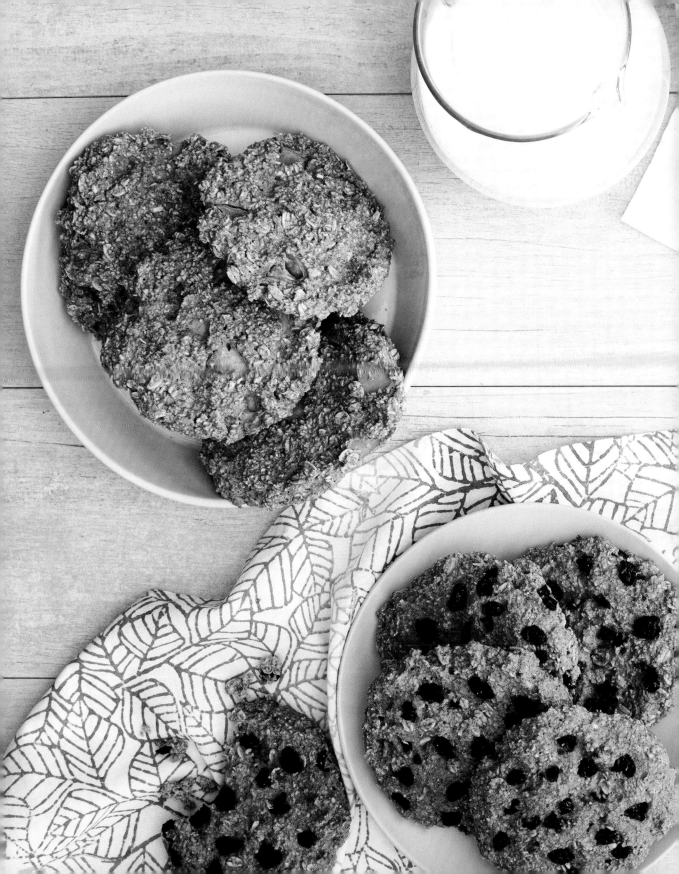

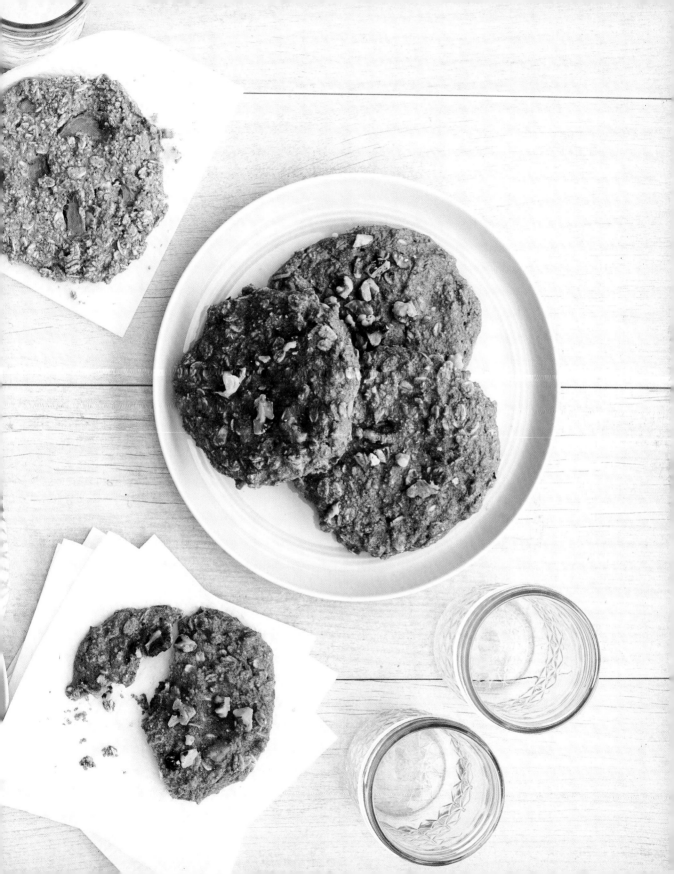

PEACH BLENDER BREAKFAST COOKIES

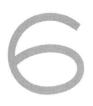 **⅙th of recipe (1 cookie):** 142 calories, 2g total fat (0.5g sat fat), 213mg sodium, 23g carbs, 3.5g fiber, 3g sugars, 8.5g protein

2 cups **old-fashioned oats**
1 cup finely chopped **peaches** (fresh or thawed from frozen; no sugar added)
½ cup (about 4 large) **egg whites** or **fat-free liquid egg substitute**
⅓ cup (about 1 standard scoop) **vanilla protein powder**
4 packets **natural no-calorie sweetener**
1½ teaspoons **baking powder**

seasonings:
2 teaspoons cinnamon
¼ teaspoon nutmeg
⅛ teaspoon salt

You'll need: baking sheet, parchment paper, blender

Prep: 15 minutes
Cook: 15 minutes

1. Preheat oven to 350 degrees. Line a baking sheet with parchment paper.

2. In a blender, pulse 1½ cups oats to the consistency of coarse flour.

3. Add ½ cup peaches, egg, protein powder, sweetener, baking powder, seasonings, and 2 tablespoons water. Blend until smooth and uniform, stopping and stirring if needed.

4. Gently fold in remaining ½ cup oats and ½ cup peaches.

5. Evenly distribute batter into 6 mounds on the baking sheet, about ⅓ cup each. With the back of a spoon, lightly flatten into 5-inch circles.

6. Bake until a knife inserted into the center of a cookie comes out clean, 10 to 12 minutes.

MAKES 6 SERVINGS

BANANA NUT BLENDER BREAKFAST COOKIES

30m **V** **GF** **⅙th of recipe (1 cookie):** 194 calories, 5g total fat (0.5g sat fat), 215mg sodium, 29g carbs, 4.5g fiber, 5.5g sugars, 9.5g protein

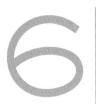

2 cups **old-fashioned oats**
1 cup (about 2 medium) mashed **extra-ripe bananas**
½ cup (about 4 large) **egg whites** or **fat-free liquid egg substitute**
⅓ cup (about 1 standard scoop) **vanilla protein powder**
1½ teaspoons **baking powder**
1 ounce (about ¼ cup) **walnuts**, chopped

seasonings:
1 tablespoon cinnamon
⅛ teaspoon salt

194 CALORIES

You'll need: baking sheet, parchment paper, blender

Prep: 15 minutes
Cook: 15 minutes

1. Preheat oven to 350 degrees. Line a baking sheet with parchment paper.

2. In a blender, pulse 1½ cups oats to the consistency of coarse flour.

3. Add banana, egg, protein powder, baking powder, and seasonings. Blend until smooth and uniform, stopping and stirring if needed.

4. Gently fold in remaining ½ cup oats and 2 tablespoons walnuts.

5. Evenly distribute batter into 6 mounds on the baking sheet, about ⅓ cup each. With the back of a spoon, lightly flatten into 5-inch circles.

6. Sprinkle with remaining 2 tablespoons walnuts, and lightly press to adhere.

7. Bake until a knife inserted into the center of a cookie comes out clean, 10 to 12 minutes.

MAKES 6 SERVINGS

BLENDER BANANA BREAD

(V) (GF) **⅛th of recipe (1 slice):** 110 calories, 1.5g total fat (<0.5g sat fat), 189mg sodium, 25g carbs, 3g fiber, 4g sugars, 4.5g protein

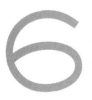

2 cups **old-fashioned oats**
1 cup (about 2 medium) mashed **extra-ripe bananas**
½ cup (about 4 large) **egg whites** or **fat-free liquid egg substitute**
¼ cup **unsweetened vanilla almond milk**
3 tablespoons **Truvia spoonable no-calorie sweetener**
2 teaspoons **baking powder**

seasonings:
½ teaspoon cinnamon
⅛ teaspoon salt

110 CALORIES

You'll need: 9-inch by 5-inch loaf pan, nonstick spray, blender

Prep: 5 minutes
Cook: 40 minutes

1. Preheat oven to 350 degrees. Spray a 9-inch by 5-inch loaf pan with nonstick spray.

2. In a blender, pulse oats to the consistency of coarse flour.

3. Add all remaining ingredients and seasonings to the blender. Blend until smooth and uniform, stopping and stirring as needed.

4. Transfer to the baking pan, and smooth out the top. Bake until a knife inserted into the center comes out clean, 35 to 40 minutes.

MAKES 8 SERVINGS

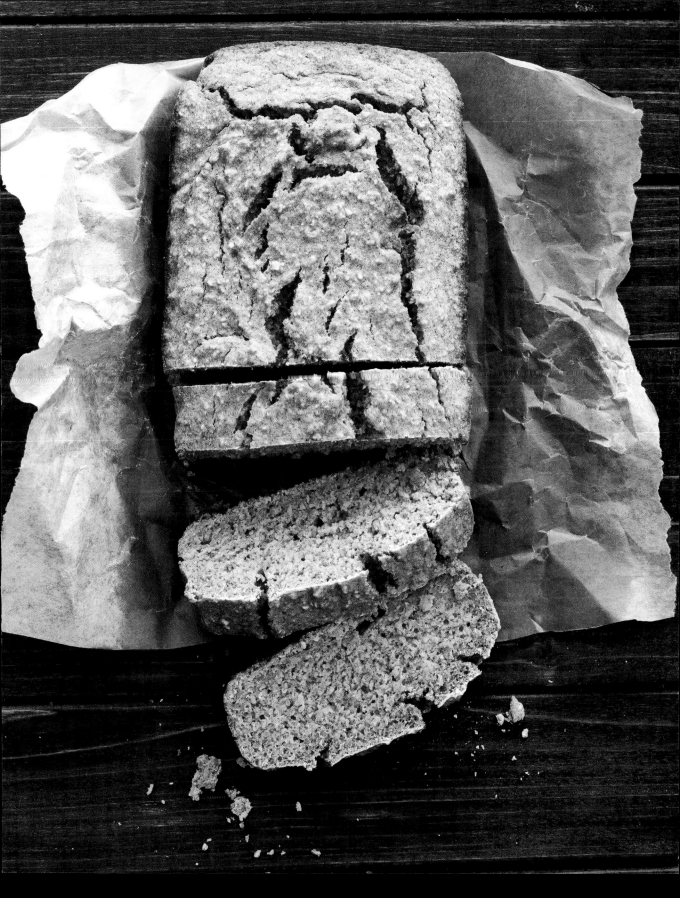

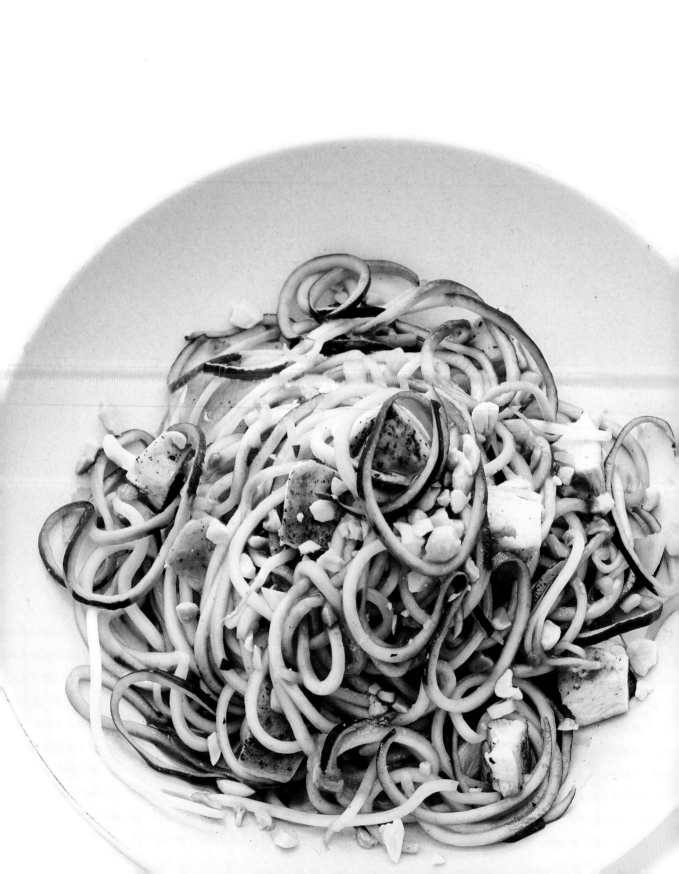

3

SIMPLY CHICKEN

Chicken is definitely one of my FAVORITE forms of lean protein, and I know I'm not alone . . . This chapter features chicken recipes made in an Instant Pot, slow cooker, foil pack, and more.

INSTANT-POT SIMPLE SHREDDED CHICKEN

 ¼th of recipe (about ⅔ cup): 144 calories, 3g total fat (0.5g sat fat), 592mg sodium, 1.5g carbs, <0.5g fiber, 1g sugars, 26g protein

2

1 pound **raw boneless skinless chicken breast**
2 cups **chicken broth**

seasonings:
1 teaspoon garlic powder
1 teaspoon onion powder
¼ teaspoon each salt and black pepper

You'll need: Instant Pot, large bowl

Prep: 5 minutes
Cook: 20 minutes

1. Place chicken in the Instant Pot, and sprinkle with seasonings.

2. Add broth. Top with lid, and seal. Press Manual, and set for 6 minutes.

3. Press Keep Warm/Cancel.

4. Vent to release steam.

5. Transfer chicken to a large bowl. (Discard broth, or save for another time.) Shred with two forks.

MAKES 4 SERVINGS

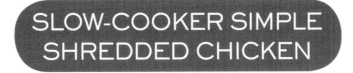

SLOW-COOKER SIMPLE SHREDDED CHICKEN

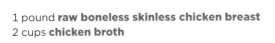

GF **¼th of recipe (about ⅔ cup):** 144 calories, 3g total fat (0.5g sat fat), 592mg sodium, 1.5g carbs, <0.5g fiber, 1g sugars, 26g protein

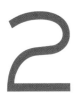

1 pound **raw boneless skinless chicken breast**
2 cups **chicken broth**

seasonings:
1 teaspoon garlic powder
1 teaspoon onion powder
¼ teaspoon each salt and black pepper

144 CALORIES

You'll need: slow cooker, large bowl

Prep: 5 minutes
Cook: 2 hours or 4 hours

1. Place chicken in a slow cooker, and sprinkle with seasonings.

2. Add broth. Cover and cook for 2 hours on high or 4 hours on low, until chicken is cooked through.

3. Transfer chicken to a large bowl. (Discard broth, or save for another time.) Shred with two forks.

MAKES 4 SERVINGS

6 SIMPLE WAYS TO SERVE SHREDDED CHICKEN

I love shredded chicken so much, I included THREE different ways to prepare it in this book. It's endlessly versatile; check it out . . .

1. **In wraps and burritos**

2. **In salad or lettuce cups**

3. **Mixed with teriyaki or BBQ sauce**

4. **Added to egg scrambles**

5. **Baked into casseroles**

6. **Stirred into slaws**

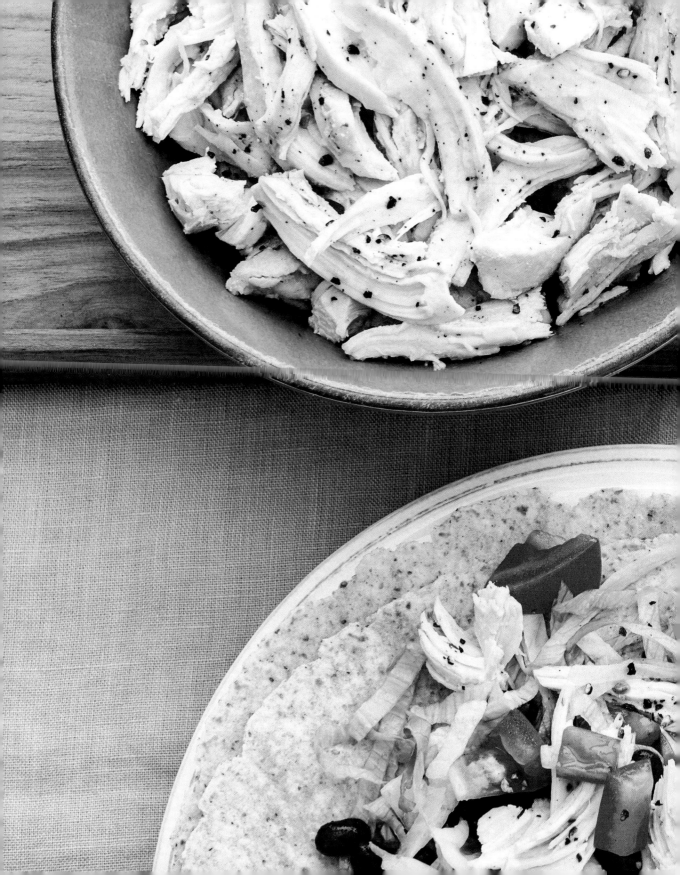

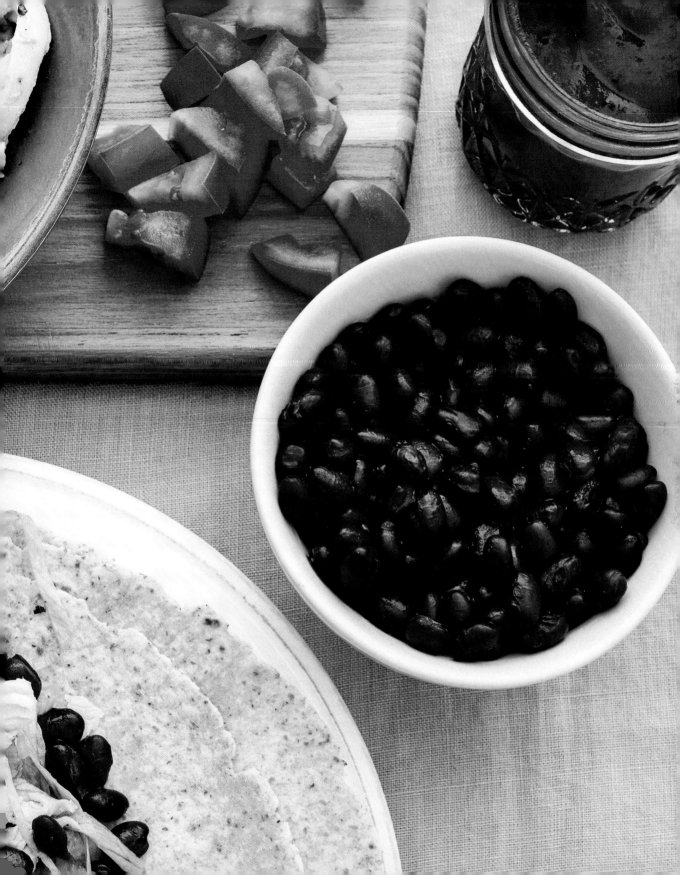

FOIL-PACK SIMPLE SHREDDED CHICKEN

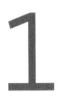 **¼th of recipe (about ⅔ cup):** 140 calories, 3g total fat (0.5g sat fat), 197mg sodium, 1g carbs, <0.5g fiber, 0.5g sugars, 25.5g protein

1 pound **raw boneless skinless chicken breast cutlets**

seasonings:
1 teaspoon garlic powder
1 teaspoon onion powder
¼ teaspoon each salt and black pepper

140 CALORIES

You'll need: heavy-duty foil, baking sheet, nonstick spray, large bowl

Prep: 5 minutes
Cook: 25 minutes

1. Preheat oven to 375 degrees. Lay a large piece of heavy-duty foil on a baking sheet, and spray with nonstick spray.

2. Place chicken on the center of the foil, and sprinkle with seasonings. Cover with another large piece of foil. Fold together and seal all four edges of the foil pieces, forming a well-sealed packet.

3. Bake for 25 minutes, or until chicken is cooked through.

4. Cut packet to release hot steam before opening entirely.

5. Transfer chicken to a large bowl. Shred with two forks.

MAKES 4 SERVINGS

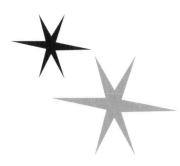

Chick Chick Hooray!

FROZEN CHICKEN BREAST IS A GREAT KITCHEN STAPLE

Defrost it by letting it thaw naturally in the fridge overnight. Crunched for time? Submerge the package in a large bowl of cold water. (If it isn't tightly sealed, place it in a resealable plastic bag.) Change the water every half hour until the chicken has thawed.

SLICE & DICE WITH EASE

Another bonus to using frozen chicken? Poultry and meats are easier to cut when they're slightly frozen. For recipes that call for sliced or chopped chicken, cut into your chicken breast before it completely thaws.

CHICKEN CUTLETS ARE TIME SAVERS

Uniform pieces help achieve evenly cooked chicken. And no one wants overcooked ends with a barely cooked middle! Your best bet is to buy chicken breast cutlets versus whole breasts. They're generally even in thickness right out of the package.

EZ FAUX-FRIED CHICKEN STRIPS

¼th of recipe (about 3 pieces): 191 calories, 3g total fat (0.5g sat fat), 367mg sodium, 9g carbs, 1g fiber, 2g sugars, 29.5g protein

½ cup **fat-free plain Greek yogurt**
1 pound (about 12 pieces) **raw boneless skinless chicken breast tenders**
½ cup **whole-wheat panko breadcrumbs**

seasonings:
¼ teaspoon paprika
1 tablespoon dried minced onion
1 teaspoon garlic powder
½ teaspoon salt
¼ teaspoon black pepper

191 CALORIES

You'll need: medium bowl, large sealable bag, baking sheet, nonstick spray, wide bowl

Prep: 15 minutes
Marinate: 1 hour
Cook: 25 minutes

1. In a medium bowl, mix yogurt with paprika.

2. Place chicken tenders in a large sealable bag, top with seasoned yogurt, and thoroughly coat. Tightly seal, removing as much air as possible. Marinate in the fridge for at least 1 hour.

3. Preheat oven to 375 degrees. Spray a baking sheet with nonstick spray.

4. In a wide bowl, mix breadcrumbs with remaining seasonings.

5. One at a time, coat chicken tenders with seasoned crumbs, first removing excess yogurt if needed.

6. Place on the baking sheet, and top with any remaining crumbs. Bake for 10 minutes.

7. Flip chicken. Bake until cooked through and crispy, 10 to 12 minutes.

MAKES 4 SERVINGS

HG FYI

If you can't find whole-wheat panko, use regular panko breadcrumbs instead. (Your chicken strips will just have a little less fiber.)

EXTRA, EXTRA!

Dip your chicken strips in BBQ sauce, honey mustard, or ketchup . . . or all three!

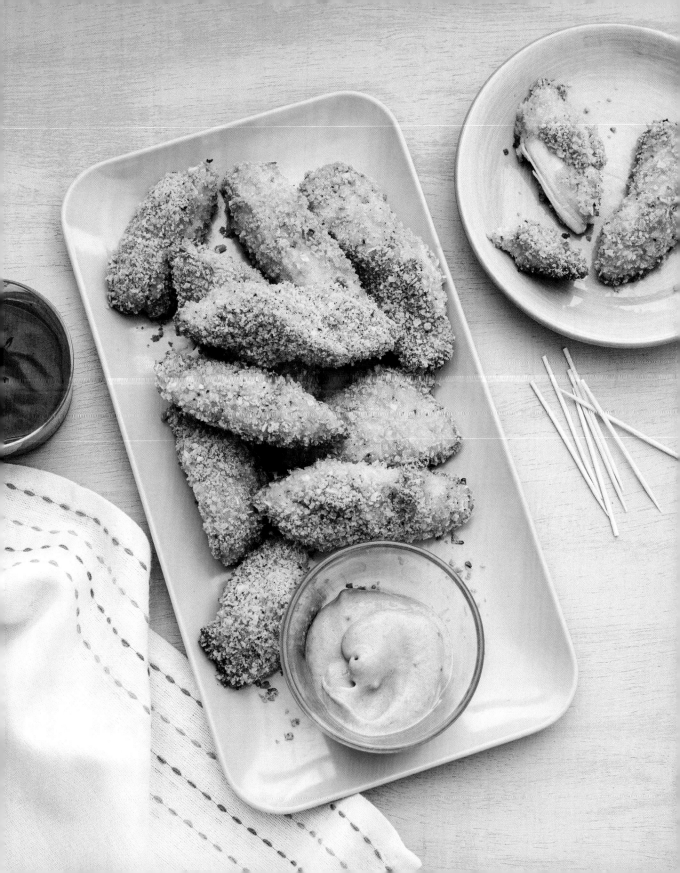

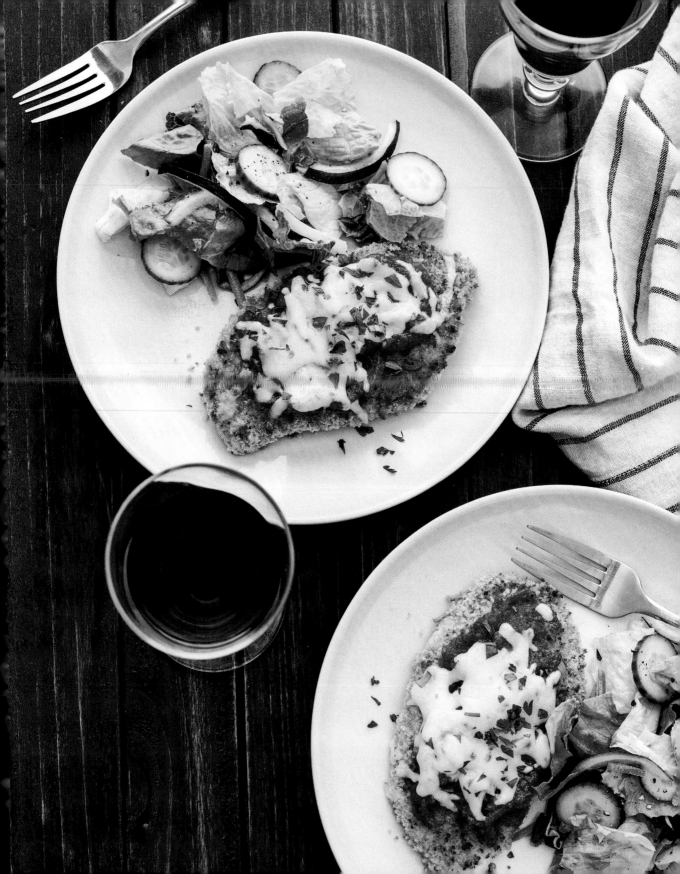

SKILLET CHICKEN PARMESAN

 **½ of recipe (1 cutlet):** 270 calories, 6.5g total fat (2.5g sat fat), 620mg sodium, 13.5g carbs, 2g fiber, 2.5g sugars, 36g protein

5

⅓ cup **whole-wheat panko breadcrumbs**
¼ cup (about 2 large) **egg whites** or **fat-free liquid egg substitute**
Two 4-ounce **raw boneless skinless chicken breast cutlets**
⅓ cup **canned crushed tomatoes**
⅓ cup shredded **part-skim mozzarella cheese**

seasonings:
¾ teaspoon Italian seasoning
¾ teaspoon garlic powder
¾ teaspoon onion powder
¼ teaspoon salt

270 CALORIES

You'll need: two wide bowls, large skillet with lid, nonstick spray, small bowl

Prep: 10 minutes
Cook: 15 minutes

1. In a wide bowl, mix breadcrumbs with ¼ teaspoon of each seasoning. Place egg in another wide bowl.

2. Season chicken with ¼ teaspoon each Italian seasoning, garlic powder, and onion powder. Coat with egg, shake to remove excess, and coat with seasoned crumbs.

3. Bring a large skillet sprayed with nonstick spray to medium heat. Cook chicken for about 4 minutes per side, until cooked through.

4. Meanwhile, in a small bowl, mix crushed tomatoes with remaining ¼ teaspoon each Italian seasoning, garlic powder, and onion powder.

5. Reduce heat to low. Top chicken with seasoned tomatoes and cheese. Cover and cook until cheese has melted, about 3 minutes.

MAKES 2 SERVINGS

SWEET & SPICY BUFFALO CHICKEN NUGGETS

30m **½ of recipe (5 nuggets):** 229 calories, 3g total fat (0.5g sat fat), 624mg sodium, 19.5g carbs, 1g fiber, 11.5g sugars, 28g protein

¼ cup **whole-wheat panko breadcrumbs**

8 ounces **raw boneless skinless chicken breast**, cut into 10 nuggets

2 tablespoons (about 1) **egg white** or **fat-free liquid egg substitute**

2 tablespoons **sweet Asian chili sauce**

1 tablespoon **Frank's RedHot Original Cayenne Pepper Sauce**

1 teaspoon **honey**

seasonings:

¼ teaspoon garlic powder

¼ teaspoon onion powder

229 CALORIES

You'll need: baking sheet, nonstick spray, two wide bowls, medium-large bowl

Prep: 10 minutes
Cook: 20 minutes

1. Preheat oven to 375 degrees. Spray a baking sheet with nonstick spray.

2. In a wide bowl, mix breadcrumbs with seasonings.

3. Place chicken in another wide bowl. Top with egg, and flip to coat.

4. One at a time, shake chicken nuggets to remove excess egg, and coat with seasoned crumbs.

5. Place on the baking sheet, and top with any remaining breadcrumbs. Bake for 8 minutes.

6. Flip chicken. Bake until light golden brown and crispy, 8 to 10 minutes.

7. Meanwhile, mix remaining ingredients in a medium-large bowl.

8. Add cooked chicken to the bowl, and gently toss to coat.

MAKES 2 SERVINGS

EXTRA, EXTRA!

Nothing says hot wings like a side of carrots, celery sticks, and (light) blue cheese dressing for dipping!

SURVEY SAYS . . .

A whopping 65% of Hungry Girl fans would choose Frank's RedHot over Tabasco. I'm with them!

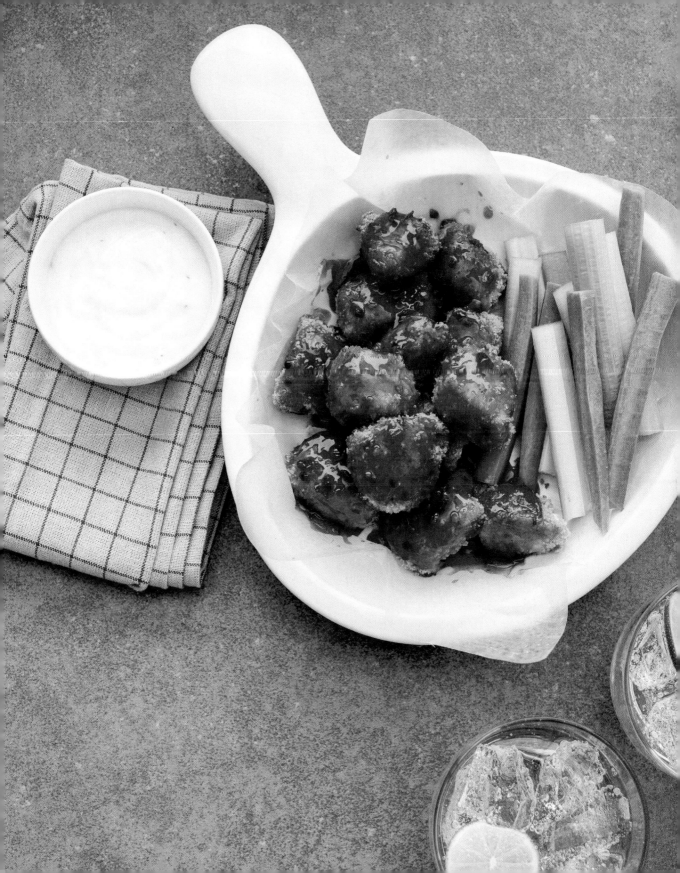

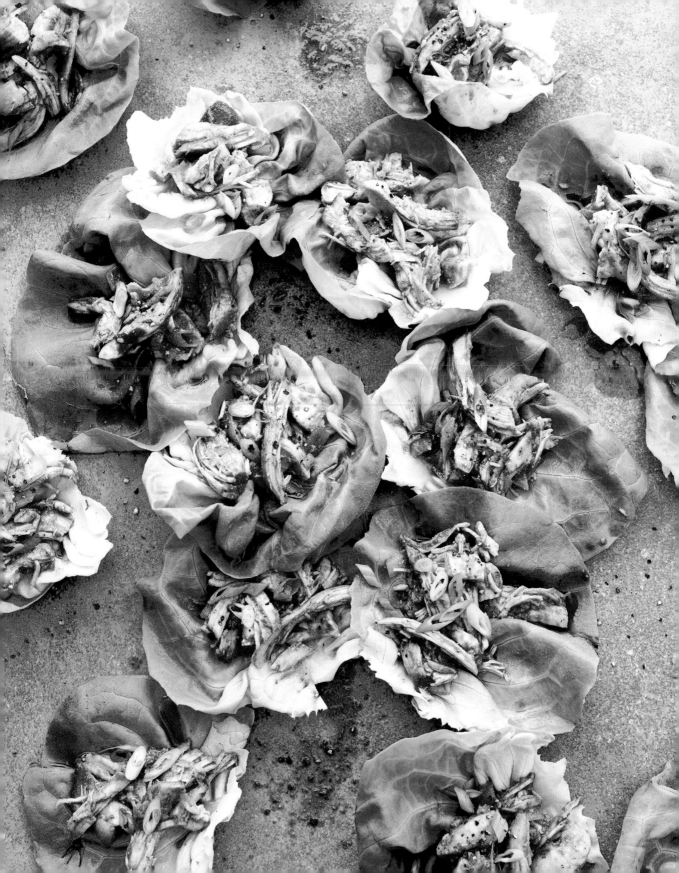

SLOW-COOKER HONEY SRIRACHA CHICKEN

 GF **⅕th of recipe (about ¾ cup):** 237 calories, 3g total fat (0.5g sat fat), 650mg sodium, 25g carbs, 0.5g fiber, 21.5g sugars, 26g protein

4

⅓ cup **honey**
⅓ cup **sriracha hot chili sauce**
1¼ pounds **raw boneless skinless chicken breast**
1 cup chopped **onion**

seasonings:
½ teaspoon garlic powder
½ teaspoon onion powder
¼ teaspoon each salt and black pepper

237 CALORIES

You'll need: slow cooker, large bowl

Prep: 5 minutes
Cook: 3 to 4 hours or 7 to 8 hours

1. In a slow cooker, combine honey, sriracha, garlic powder, and onion powder. Stir until uniform.

2. Season chicken with salt and pepper, and add to the slow cooker.

3. Top with onion. Cover and cook on high for 3 to 4 hours or on low for 7 to 8 hours, until chicken is fully cooked.

4. Transfer chicken to a large bowl. Shred with two forks.

5. Return chicken to the slow cooker, and mix well.

MAKES 5 SERVINGS

EXTRA, EXTRA!

Skip the starchy carbs . . . Serve this up in lettuce cups, and top it off with scallions.

SLOW-COOKER CHICKEN VEGGIE SOUP

GF **⅛th of recipe (about 1 heaping cup):** 116 calories, 2g total fat (0.5g sat fat), 540mg sodium, 5.5g carbs, 1g fiber, 2.5g sugars, 17g protein

1¼ pounds **raw boneless skinless chicken breast**
6 cups **reduced-sodium chicken broth**
1½ cups sliced **carrots**
1 cup chopped **celery**
1 cup chopped **onion**
2 teaspoons chopped **garlic**

seasonings:
¼ teaspoon each salt and black pepper
½ teaspoon onion powder
½ teaspoon ground thyme

116 CALORIES

You'll need: slow cooker, large bowl

Prep: 10 minutes
Cook: 3 to 4 hours or 7 to 8 hours

1. Place chicken in a slow cooker, and season with salt and pepper. Add remaining ingredients and seasonings, and mix well.

2. Cover and cook on high for 3 to 4 hours or on low for 7 to 8 hours, until chicken is fully cooked.

3. Transfer chicken to a large bowl. Shred with two forks.

4. Return chicken to the slow cooker, and mix well.

MAKES 8 SERVINGS

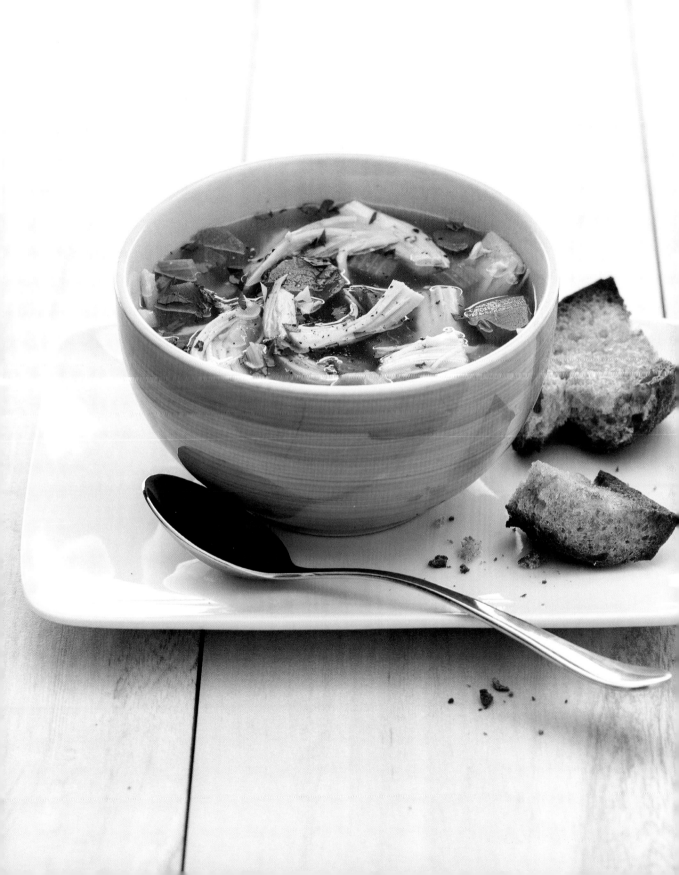

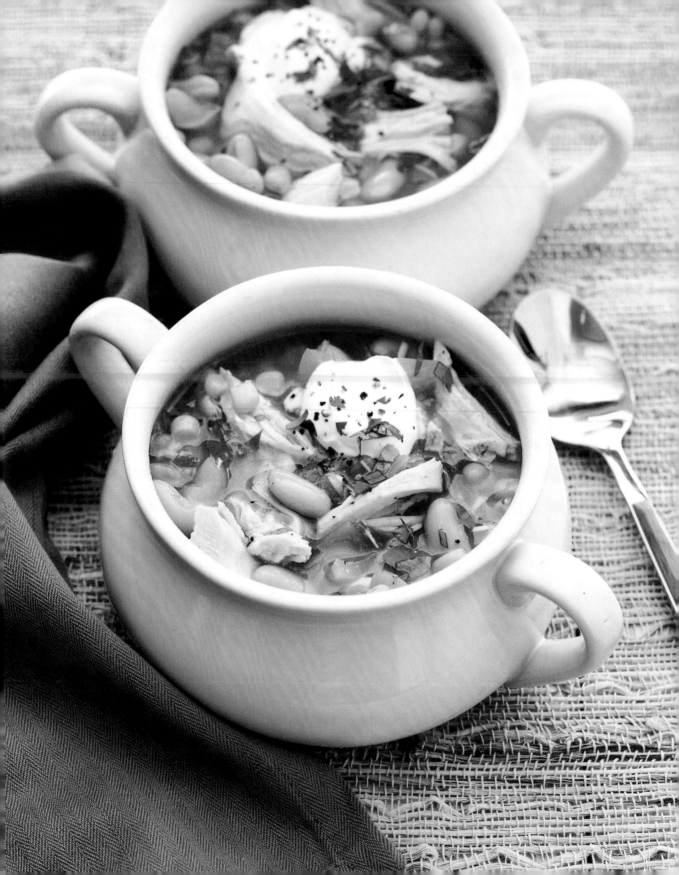

SLOW-COOKER CHICKEN CHILI STEW

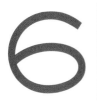

GF **⅛th of recipe (about 1 cup):** 223 calories, 2.5g total fat (0.5g sat fat), 704mg sodium, 25g carbs, 6g fiber, 4g sugars, 23.5g protein

1¼ pounds **raw boneless skinless chicken breast**
4 cups **reduced-sodium chicken broth**
Two 15.5-ounce cans **cannellini (white kidney) beans**, drained and rinsed
One 7-ounce can **diced green chiles** (not drained)
1½ cups chopped **onion**
1 cup **frozen sweet corn kernels**

seasonings:
4½ teaspoons chili seasoning
⅛ teaspoon salt

223 CALORIES

You'll need: slow cooker, large bowl

Prep: 10 minutes
Cook: 3 to 4 hours or 7 to 8 hours

1. Place chicken in a slow cooker, and season with ½ teaspoon chili seasoning.

2. Add broth, beans, chiles, onion, corn, remaining 4 teaspoons chili seasoning, and salt. Stir to mix.

3. Cover and cook on high for 3 to 4 hours or on low for 7 to 8 hours, until chicken is fully cooked.

4. Transfer chicken to a large bowl. Shred with two forks.

5. Return chicken to the slow cooker, and mix well.

MAKES 8 SERVINGS

EXTRA, EXTRA!

Top off your stew with a dollop of light sour cream!

HG FYI

**Chili seasoning is such a timesaver. Rather DIY?
Flip to page 357 for a recipe!**

ONE-POT CHICKEN CACCIATORE

 **¼th of recipe (about 1¼ cups):** 233 calories, 3g total fat (0.5g sat fat), 509mg sodium, 20.5g carbs, 5.5g fiber, 9.5g sugars, 30g protein

6

1 pound **raw boneless skinless chicken breast**, cut into bite-sized pieces
2 cups chopped **green bell peppers**
2 cups sliced **mushrooms**
1 cup chopped **onion**
1½ tablespoons chopped **garlic**
2½ cups **canned crushed tomatoes**

seasonings:
¼ teaspoon each salt and black pepper
1 teaspoon Italian seasoning
1 teaspoon onion powder

233 CALORIES

You'll need: large pot, nonstick spray

Prep: 15 minutes
Cook: 15 minutes

1. Bring a large pot sprayed with nonstick spray to medium-high heat. Add chicken, salt, and black pepper. Cook and stir for 3 minutes.

2. Add bell peppers, mushrooms, onion, and garlic. Cook and stir until veggies have softened and chicken has fully cooked, about 10 minutes.

3. Add tomatoes and remaining seasonings. Cook and stir until hot, about 2 minutes.

MAKES 4 SERVINGS

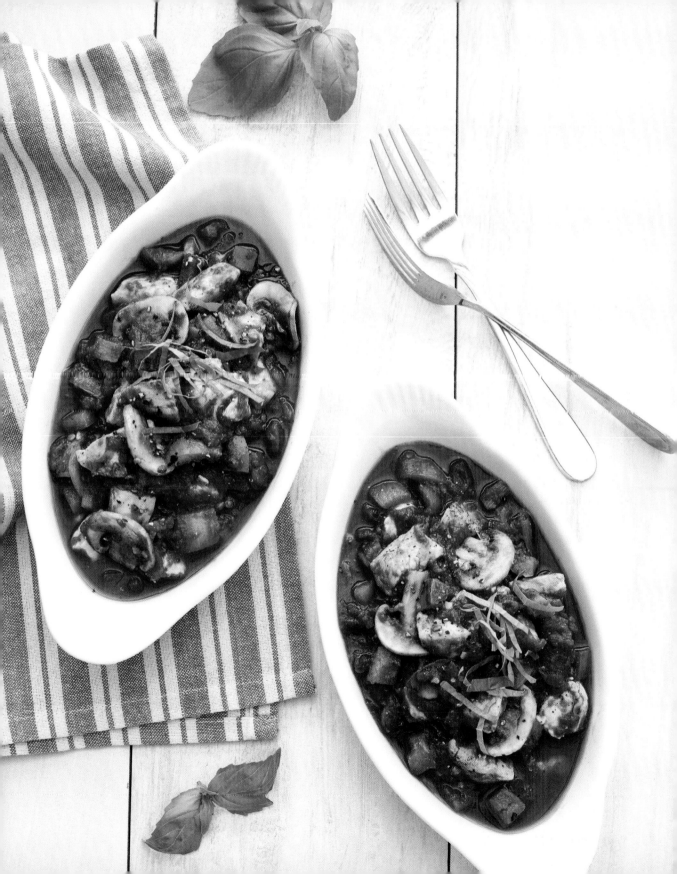

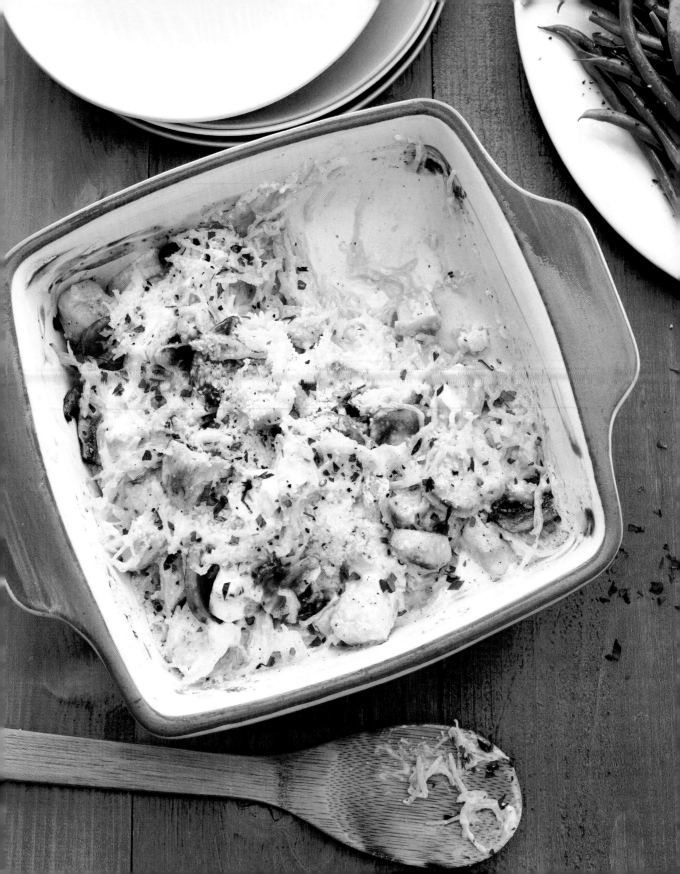

SPAGHETTI SQUASH CHICKEN TETRAZZINI

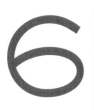 **GF** **¼th of recipe:** 278 calories, 11g total fat (5g sat fat), 614mg sodium, 18g carbs, 3g fiber, 9.5g sugars, 27.5g protein

12 ounces **raw boneless skinless chicken breast**, cut into bite-sized pieces
2 cups sliced **mushrooms**
½ cup **light sour cream**
¼ cup **light/reduced-fat cream cheese**
5 cups **cooked spaghetti squash**, drained of excess moisture
¼ cup grated **Parmesan cheese**

seasonings:
½ teaspoon each salt and black pepper
2 teaspoons dried minced onion
½ teaspoon garlic powder

278 CALORIES

You'll need: 8-inch by 8-inch baking pan, nonstick spray, skillet, large bowl

Prep: 15 minutes
Cook: 25 minutes

Plus prep and cook times for spaghetti squash (pages 241–243) if not made in advance.

1. Preheat oven to 375 degrees. Spray an 8-inch by 8-inch baking pan with nonstick spray.

2. Bring a skillet sprayed with nonstick spray to medium-high heat. Add chicken, mushrooms, and ¼ teaspoon each salt and pepper. Cook and stir for about 6 minutes, until chicken has fully cooked and mushrooms have softened.

3. Add sour cream, cream cheese, and remaining seasonings, including remaining ¼ teaspoon each salt and pepper. Cook and stir until cream cheese has melted and sauce is uniform, about 1 minute.

4. Place spaghetti squash in a large bowl. Add contents of the skillet, and stir to coat.

5. Transfer to the baking pan, and smooth out the top.

6. Sprinkle with Parm. Bake until hot and bubbly, about 15 minutes.

MAKES 4 SERVINGS

EASY-PEASY PEANUT ZUCCHINI NOODLES WITH CHICKEN

30m **½ of recipe (about 1¾ cups noodles with 2½ ounces chicken):** 335 calories, 11.5g total fat (1.5g sat fat), 864mg sodium, 31g carbs, 5g fiber, 20.5g sugars, 29g protein

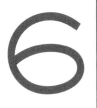

6 ounces **raw boneless skinless chicken breast cutlets**
1 pound (about 2 medium) **spiralized zucchini**
1 cup **bean sprouts**
½ cup **Thai peanut sauce or salad dressing** with 65 calories or less per 2-tablespoon serving
½ cup **canned water chestnuts**, drained and roughly chopped
4 teaspoons crushed **peanuts**

seasonings:
⅛ teaspoon each salt and black pepper

335 CALORIES

You'll need: large skillet, nonstick spray, medium bowl, strainer

Prep: 5 minutes
Cook: 15 minutes

HG FYI

Use store-bought zucchini noodles, or DIY! Flip to page 362 for the 411.

1. Season chicken with salt and pepper. Bring a large skillet sprayed with nonstick spray to medium heat. Cook for about 4 minutes per side, until cooked through. Transfer to a medium bowl.

2. Remove skillet from heat; clean, if needed. Respray, and bring to medium-high heat. Add zucchini and bean sprouts. Cook and stir until hot and slightly softened, about 3 minutes.

3. Transfer veggies to a strainer, and thoroughly drain.

4. Respray skillet and return to medium-high heat. Add drained veggies, sauce/dressing, chopped water chestnuts, and 2 teaspoons peanuts. Cook and stir until hot and uniform, about 2 minutes.

5. Chop chicken into bite-sized pieces and stir into zucchini mixture. Top with remaining 2 teaspoons peanuts.

MAKES 2 SERVINGS

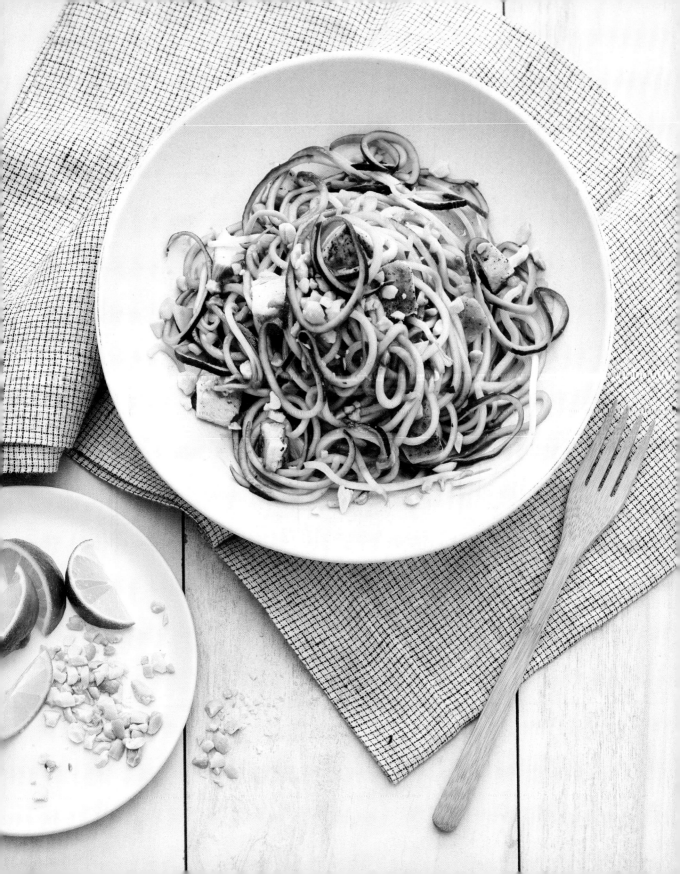

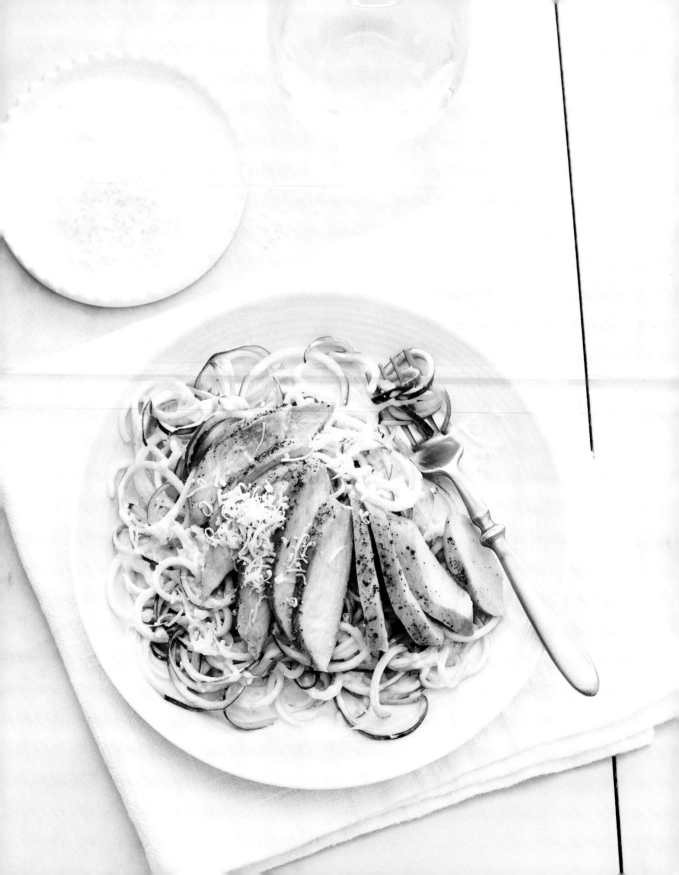

Z'PAGHETTI GIRLFREDO WITH CHICKEN

 ½ of recipe (about 1½ cups noodles with 3 ounces chicken): 309 calories, 13.5g total fat (6.5g sat fat), 740mg sodium, 14.5g carbs, 3.5g fiber, 10g sugars, 34g protein

6

8 ounces **raw boneless skinless chicken breast cutlets**
1½ pounds (about 3 medium) **spiralized zucchini**
3 tablespoons **light/reduced-fat cream cheese**
1 tablespoon **whipped butter**
2 teaspoons chopped **garlic**
4 teaspoons grated **Parmesan cheese**

seasonings:
¼ teaspoon plus ⅛ teaspoon each salt and black pepper
1 teaspoon onion powder

You'll need: extra-large skillet, nonstick spray, strainer

Prep: 5 minutes
Cook: 15 minutes

1. Bring an extra-large skillet sprayed with nonstick spray to medium heat. Season chicken with ⅛ teaspoon each salt and pepper. Cook chicken for about 4 minutes per side, until cooked through.

2. Set chicken aside. Remove skillet from heat; clean, if needed. Respray, and bring to medium-high heat. Cook and stir zucchini until hot and slightly softened, about 3 minutes.

3. Transfer zucchini to a strainer, and thoroughly drain.

4. Remove skillet from heat, respray, and bring to low heat. Add drained zucchini, cream cheese, butter, garlic, onion powder, 2 teaspoons Parm, and remaining ¼ teaspoon each salt and pepper. Cook and stir until sauce is uniform and has coated the zucchini, about 2 minutes.

5. Slice chicken, and serve over zucchini. Top with remaining 2 teaspoons Parm.

MAKES 2 SERVINGS

CAULIFLOWER ARROZ CON POLLO

GF **½ of recipe (about 2½ cups):** 290 calories, 4.5g total fat (1g sat fat), 647mg sodium, 24.5g carbs, 7.5g fiber, 10g sugars, 38.5g protein

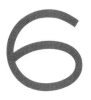

3 cups **riced cauliflower**
10 ounces **raw boneless skinless chicken breast**, cut into bite-sized pieces
¾ cup chopped **onion**
¾ cup **frozen peas and carrots**
½ cup **chicken broth**
1 tablespoon **tomato paste**

seasonings:
½ teaspoon dried oregano
¼ teaspoon ground cumin
⅛ teaspoon ground turmeric
¼ teaspoon each salt and black pepper
½ teaspoon garlic powder

You'll need: large bowl, large skillet with lid, nonstick spray, medium bowl

Prep: 10 minutes
Cook: 25 minutes

HG FYI

Use store-bought riced cauliflower, or DIY! Flip to page 365 for the 411.

1. In a large bowl, mix cauliflower, oregano, cumin, and turmeric.

2. Bring a large skillet sprayed with nonstick spray to medium heat. Season chicken with ⅛ teaspoon each salt and pepper. Cook and stir for about 5 minutes, until fully cooked. Transfer to a medium bowl.

3. Remove skillet from heat; clean, if needed. Respray, and bring to medium-high heat. Cook and stir onion until mostly softened, about 4 minutes.

4. Add seasoned cauliflower, frozen veggies, broth, tomato paste, garlic powder, and remaining ⅛ teaspoon each salt and pepper. Bring to a boil.

5. Reduce to a simmer. Cover and cook for 6 minutes.

6. Add chicken, and cook and stir until cauliflower rice is tender and chicken is hot, about 3 minutes.

MAKES 2 SERVINGS

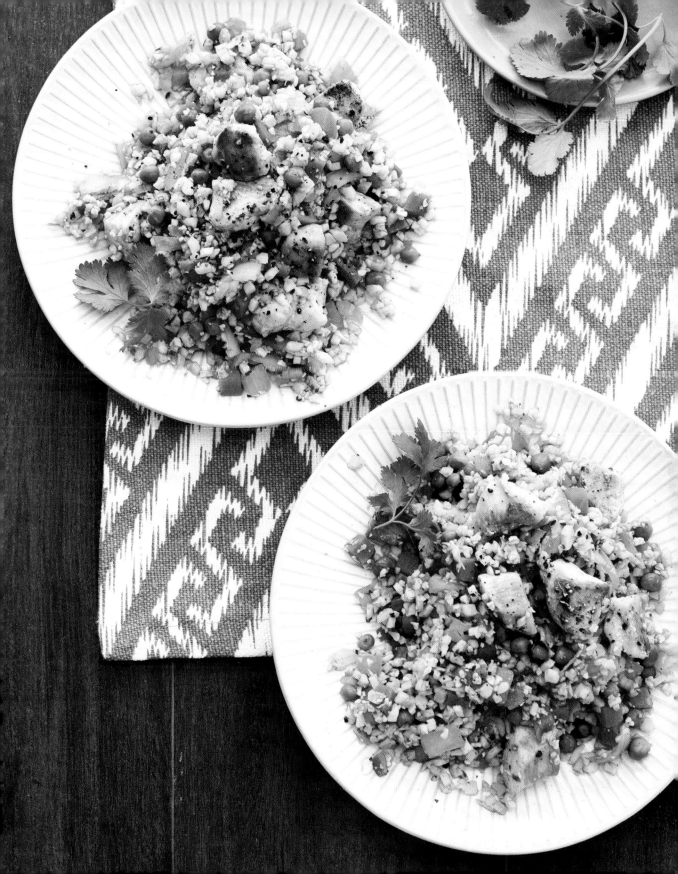

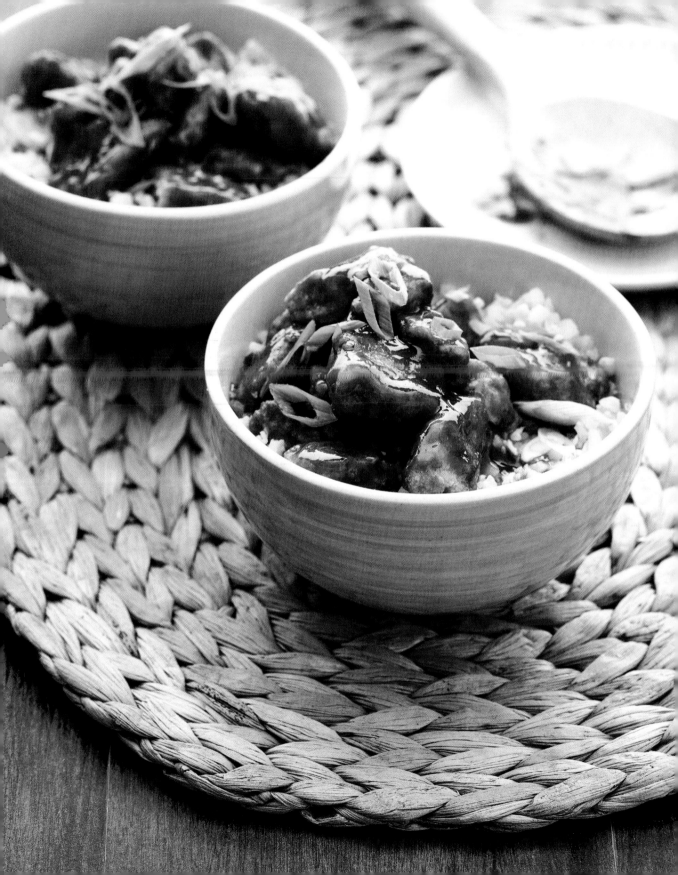

ORANGE CHICKEN

½ of recipe (about 1 cup): 279 calories, 4g total fat (0.5g sat fat), 729mg sodium, 21g carbs, 1.5g fiber, 8.5g sugars, 37g protein

3 tablespoons **whole-wheat flour**
10 ounces **raw boneless skinless chicken breast**, cut into bite-sized pieces
¼ cup (about 2 large) **egg whites** or **fat-free liquid egg substitute**
¼ cup **orange juice**
3 tablespoons **thick teriyaki sauce or marinade**
2 tablespoons chopped **scallions**

seasonings:
½ teaspoon garlic powder
¼ teaspoon ground ginger

279 CALORIES

You'll need: baking sheet, nonstick spray, two wide bowls, microwave-safe bowl, medium-large bowl

Prep: 15 minutes
Cook: 20 minutes

1. Preheat oven to 375 degrees. Spray a baking sheet with nonstick spray.

2. In a wide bowl, combine 2½ tablespoons flour, ¼ teaspoon garlic powder, and ⅛ teaspoon ground ginger. Mix well.

3. Place chicken in another wide bowl, and coat with egg.

4. One at a time, shake chicken pieces to remove excess egg and coat with flour.

5. Place on the baking sheet, and bake for 8 minutes.

6. Flip chicken. Bake until lightly browned and cooked through, about 8 more minutes.

7. Meanwhile, in a microwave-safe bowl, combine orange juice with remaining ½ tablespoon flour. Whisk with a fork to dissolve. Add teriyaki, remaining ¼ teaspoon garlic powder, and remaining ⅛ teaspoon ground ginger. Mix well. Cover and microwave for 1 minute, or until hot and thickened.

8. Place chicken in a medium-large bowl. Top with sauce, and gently toss to coat.

9. Top with scallions.

MAKES 2 SERVINGS

EXTRA, EXTRA!

Try this over cauliflower rice for a super-filling meal.

CHICKEN POT PIE STIR-FRY

30m **½ of recipe (about 1¼ cups):** 299 calories, 6g total fat (2g sat fat), 695mg sodium, 23.5g carbs, 4g fiber, 5g sugars, 33.5g protein

¼ cup **whole-wheat panko breadcrumbs**
2 tablespoons grated **Parmesan cheese**
8 ounces **raw boneless skinless chicken breast**, cut into bite-sized pieces
2 cups **frozen petite mixed vegetables**
½ cup **chicken or turkey gravy**
1 teaspoon chopped **garlic**

seasonings:
⅛ teaspoon plus a dash each salt and black pepper

299 CALORIES

You'll need: large skillet, nonstick spray, medium bowl

Prep: 5 minutes
Cook: 15 minutes

1. Bring a large skillet sprayed with nonstick spray to medium heat. Add breadcrumbs, Parm, and a dash each salt and pepper. Cook and stir until crispy and browned, about 2 minutes. Transfer to a medium bowl.

2. Remove skillet from heat, respray, and bring to medium heat. Add chicken and remaining ⅛ teaspoon each salt and pepper. Cook and stir until outside is no longer pink, about 4 minutes.

3. Add frozen veggies. Cook and stir for about 4 minutes, until veggies have thawed, excess water has evaporated, and chicken is fully cooked.

4. Add gravy and garlic. Cook and stir until hot and well mixed, about 2 minutes.

5. Top with breadcrumb mixture.

MAKES 2 SERVINGS

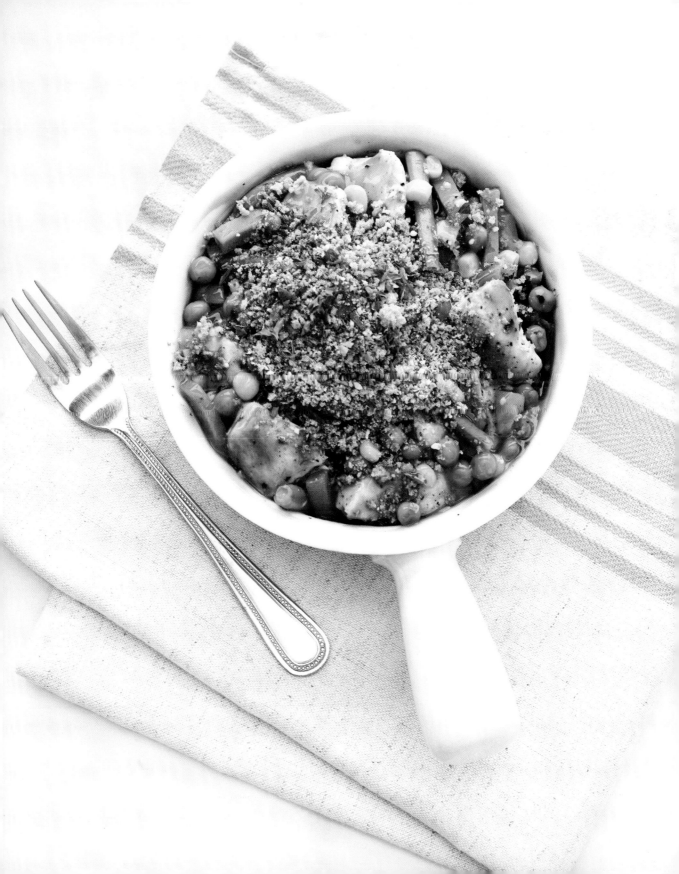

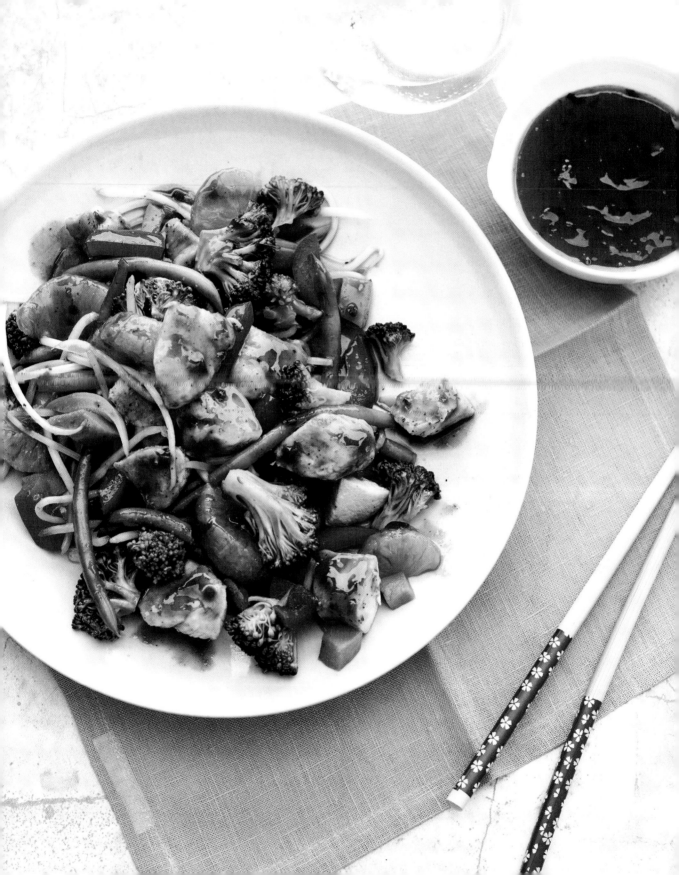

CHICKEN TERIYAKI STIR-FRY

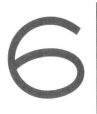

30m **½ of recipe (about 1¾ cups):** 286 calories, 3.5g total fat (0.5g sat fat), 767mg sodium, 31.5g carbs, 5g fiber, 21.5g sugars, 30.5g protein

6

2 tablespoons **thick teriyaki sauce or marinade**
1 tablespoon **sweet Asian chili sauce**
8 ounces **raw boneless skinless chicken breast**, cut into bite-sized pieces
3 cups frozen **Asian-style stir-fry vegetables**
1½ cups **bean sprouts**
½ cup **mandarin orange segments** packed in juice (not drained)

seasonings:
¼ teaspoon ground ginger
¼ teaspoon garlic powder
⅛ teaspoon each salt and black pepper

286 CALORIES

You'll need: small bowl, wok (or large skillet), nonstick spray

Prep: 10 minutes
Cook: 10 minutes

1. In a small bowl, combine teriyaki sauce, chili sauce, ginger, and 1 tablespoon water. Mix well.

2. Bring a wok (or large skillet) sprayed with nonstick spray to medium-high heat. Add chicken, and sprinkle with remaining seasonings.

3. Add frozen veggies and bean sprouts. Cook and stir for about 5 minutes, until chicken is cooked through and veggies are hot and tender.

4. Add sauce mixture and mandarin orange segments. Cook and stir until hot and well mixed, about 2 minutes.

MAKES 2 SERVINGS

SHEET-PAN CHICKEN FAJITAS

 **GF** **½ of recipe (about 1½ cups):** 229 calories, 7.5g total fat (1g sat fat), 200mg sodium, 12g carbs, 3g fiber, 5.5g sugars, 27g protein

6

2 teaspoons **olive oil**
1½ teaspoons **lime juice**
8 ounces **raw boneless skinless chicken breast**, cut into strips
2 cups sliced **bell peppers**
1 cup sliced **onion**
2 tablespoons chopped **fresh cilantro**

seasonings:
2 teaspoons taco seasoning

You'll need: baking sheet, nonstick spray, large bowl

Prep: 10 minutes
Cook: 20 minutes

1. Preheat oven to 400 degrees. Spray a baking sheet with nonstick spray.

2. In a large bowl, use a fork to whisk oil with lime juice. Add chicken, veggies, and seasoning, and toss to coat.

3. Transfer to the baking sheet. Bake for 10 minutes.

4. Flip/rearrange chicken and veggies. Bake until chicken is cooked through and veggies are tender, about 10 minutes.

5. Top with cilantro.

MAKES 2 SERVINGS

HG FYI

DIY taco seasoning! Find it on page 358.

EXTRA, EXTRA!

There are so many ways to serve this one . . . I love it in corn tortillas or lettuce wraps with salsa, light sour cream, and hot sauce.

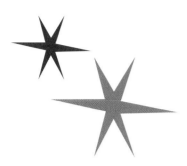

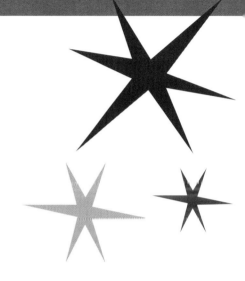

Hungry for More Mexican Food?

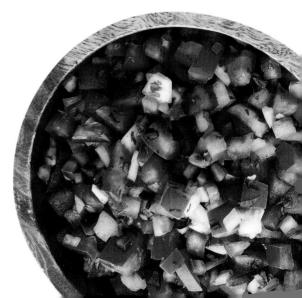

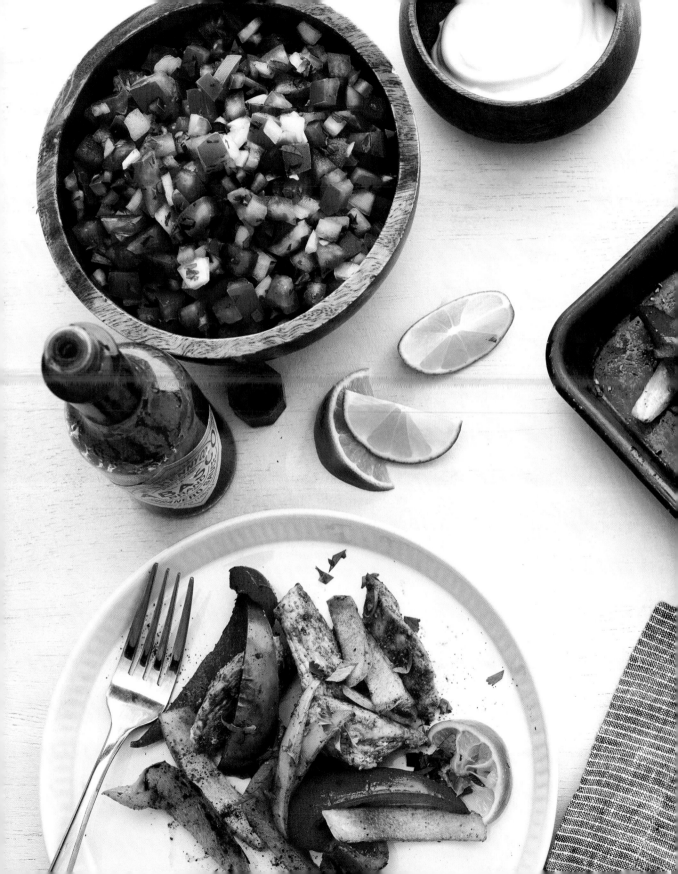

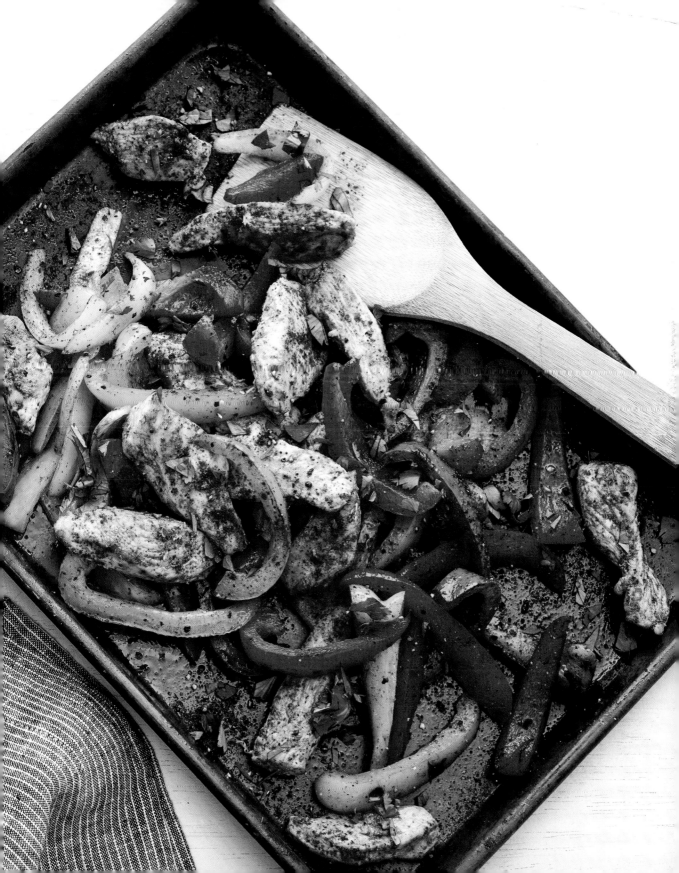

EZ BBQ CHICKEN QUESADILLA

Entire recipe: 325 calories, 10g total fat (4.5g sat fat), 752mg sodium, 32.5g carbs, 6.5g fiber, 6g sugars, 32g protein

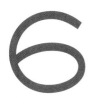

One 3-ounce **raw boneless skinless chicken breast cutlet**
1 tablespoon **BBQ sauce** with 45 calories or less per 2-tablespoon serving, or more for topping
1 **large high-fiber flour tortilla** with 110 calories or less
¼ cup shredded **reduced-fat Mexican-blend cheese**
2 tablespoons chopped **red onion**
1 tablespoon chopped **fresh cilantro**

seasonings:
⅛ teaspoon garlic powder
⅛ teaspoon onion powder

325 CALORIES

You'll need: skillet, nonstick spray, small bowl

Prep: 5 minutes
Cook: 15 minutes

1. Bring a skillet sprayed with nonstick spray to medium-high heat. Sprinkle chicken with seasonings, and cook for about 4 minutes per side, until cooked through.

2. Once cool enough to handle, roughly chop. In a small bowl, coat chicken with BBQ sauce.

3. Lay tortilla flat, and spread BBQ chicken onto one half. Top chicken with remaining ingredients.

4. Clean skillet, if needed. Respray and return to medium-high heat. Cook the half-loaded tortilla for 2 minutes.

5. Fold the bare tortilla half over the filling with a spatula, and press lightly to seal. Carefully flip and cook until crispy, about 3 minutes.

6. Slice into wedges.

MAKES 1 SERVING

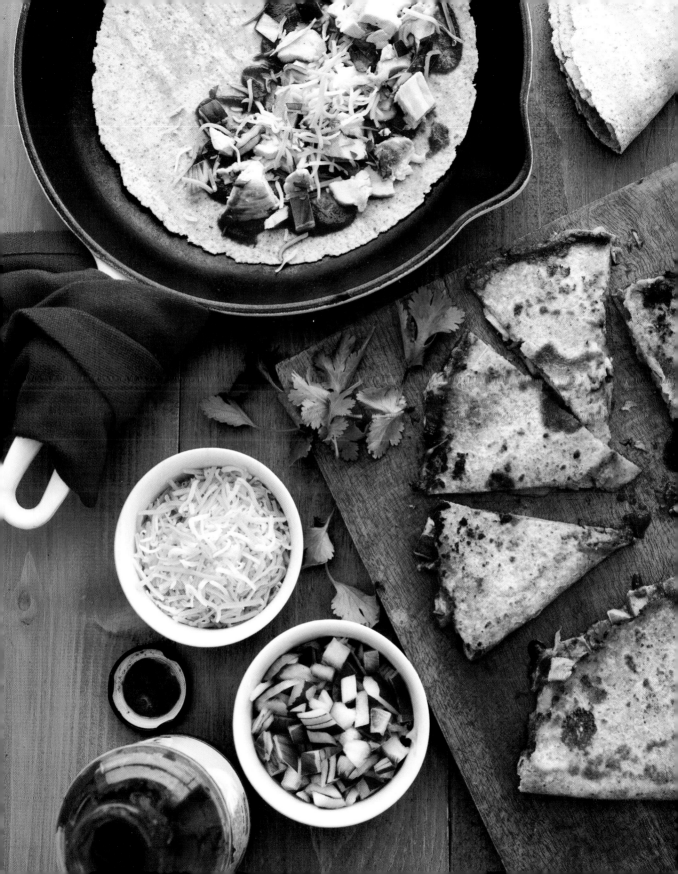

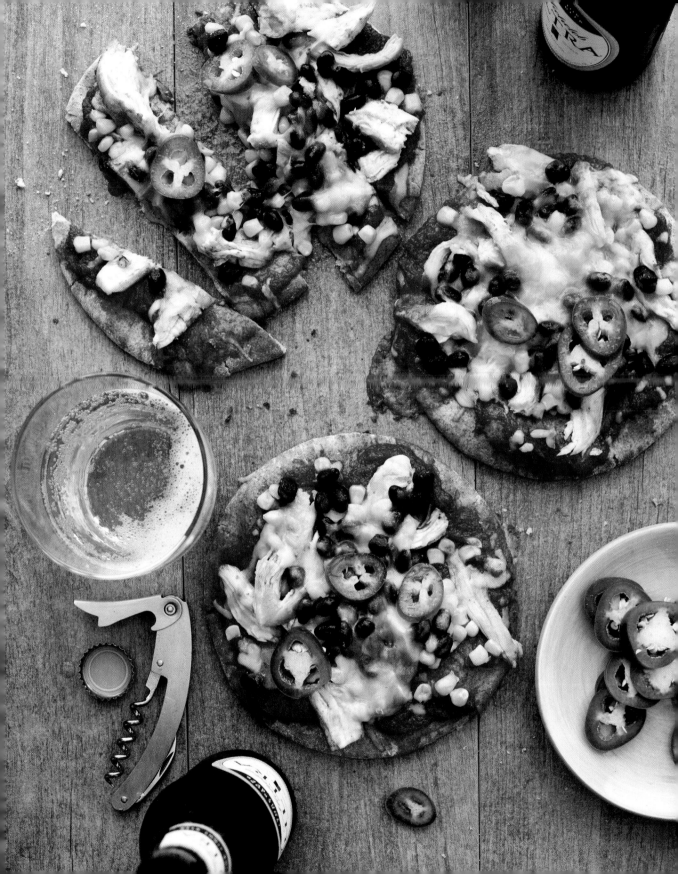

SOUTHWEST CHICKEN PITA PIZZA

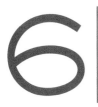 **Entire recipe:** 374 calories, 9.5g total fat (4g sat fat), 767mg sodium, 41.5g carbs, 9g fiber, 4.5g sugars, 36g protein

6

One 3-ounce **raw boneless skinless chicken breast cutlet**
¼ cup **canned crushed tomatoes**
1 **whole-wheat pita**
¼ cup shredded **reduced-fat Mexican-blend cheese**
2 tablespoons **frozen sweet corn kernels**
1½ tablespoons **canned black beans**, drained and rinsed

seasonings:
¼ teaspoon onion powder
¼ teaspoon ground cumin
¼ teaspoon chili powder

You'll need: baking sheet, nonstick spray, skillet, small bowl

Prep: 10 minutes
Cook: 20 minutes

1. Preheat oven to 375 degrees. Spray a baking sheet with nonstick spray.

2. Bring a skillet sprayed with nonstick spray to medium heat. Sprinkle chicken with ⅛ teaspoon of each seasoning, and cook for about 4 minutes per side, until cooked through.

3. Once cool enough to handle, roughly chop.

4. In a small bowl, mix tomatoes with remaining ⅛ teaspoon of each seasoning.

5. Place pita on the baking sheet, and spread with seasoned tomatoes, leaving a ½-inch border. Top with chicken and remaining ingredients.

6. Bake until hot and lightly browned, 10 to 12 minutes.

MAKES 1 SERVING

EXTRA, EXTRA!

Like things hot? Add sliced jalapeño . . . but keep a glass of water nearby!

HEY, POULTRY LOVERS!

Check out the ground beef recipes in the next chapter. Why? Because they can be made with ground turkey instead!

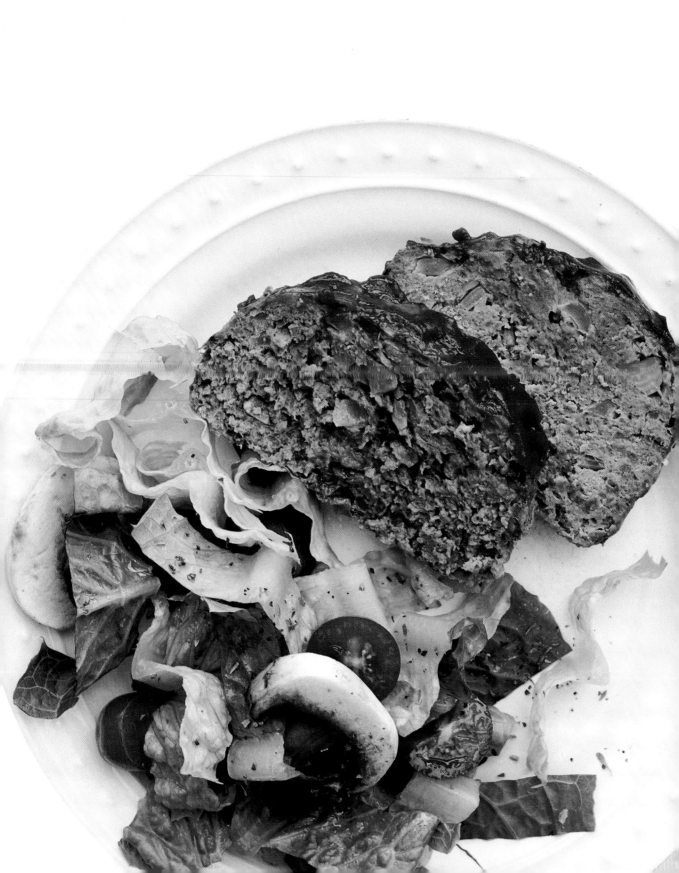

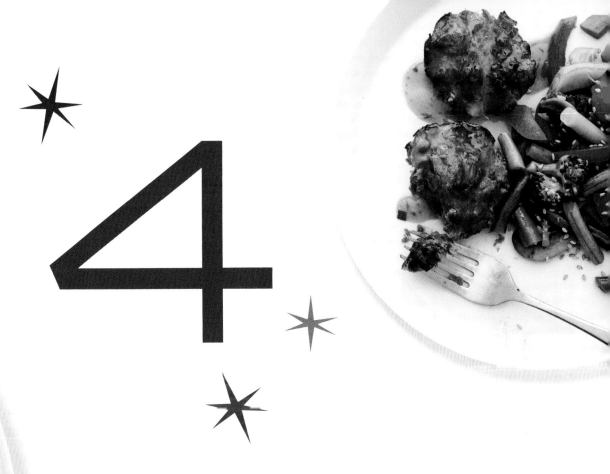

4

SIMPLY BEEF (& PORK)

Calling all meat lovers! This chapter serves up comfort-food classics and brand-new creations. Plus, the go-to ground beef recipe you'll use again and again . . .

SUPER-SIZED GROUND BEEF

 ¼th of recipe (about 1 cup): 169 calories, 5g total fat (2g sat fat), 220mg sodium, 5g carbs, 1g fiber, 2.5g sugars, 25g protein

3

1 pound **raw extra-lean ground beef**
2 cups finely chopped **mushrooms**
1 cup finely chopped **onion**

seasonings:
¼ teaspoon garlic powder
¼ teaspoon salt
⅛ teaspoon black pepper

169 CALORIES

You'll need: large skillet, nonstick spray

Prep: 10 minutes
Cook: 10 minutes

1. Bring a large skillet sprayed with nonstick spray to medium-high heat. Add all ingredients and seasonings. Cook and crumble for 6 to 8 minutes, until beef is fully cooked and veggies have softened.

2. Drain excess liquid, if needed.

MAKES 4 SERVINGS

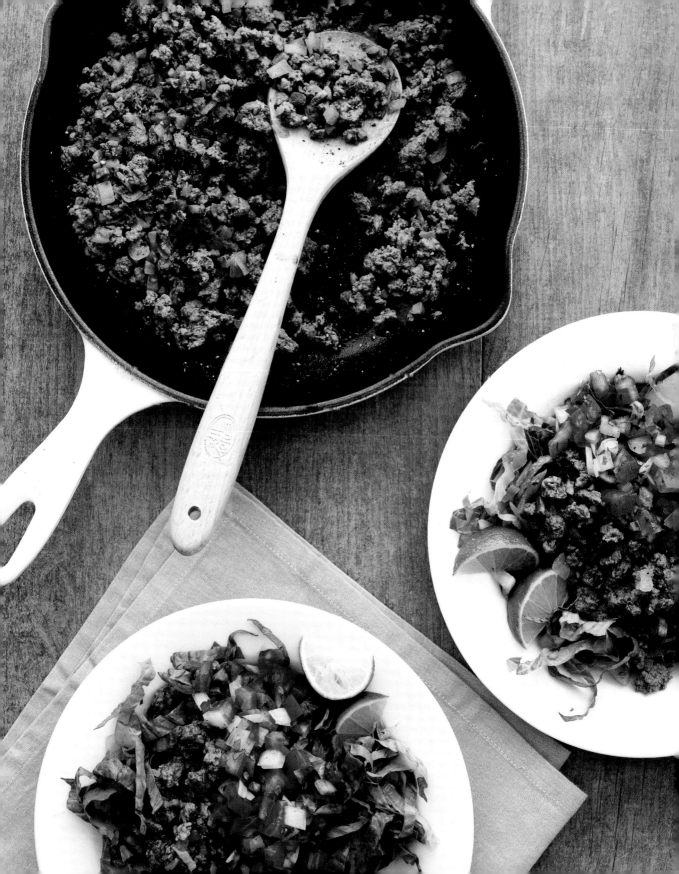

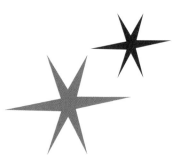

6 Simple Ways to Serve Super-Sized Ground Beef

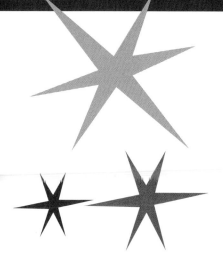

1. On a salad with salsa

2. In tacos (hard or soft!)

3. Over shredded lettuce with burger fixins

4. With frozen stir-fry veggies and teriyaki

5. Over cauliflower rice with gravy

6. With marinara over veggie noodles

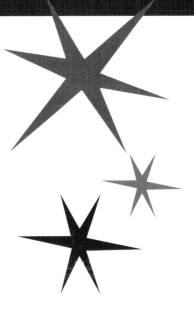

Beef vs. Turkey

Ground Hero!

You might be wondering why these recipes call for ground beef and not ground turkey. Extra-lean ground beef actually has a lot going for it! It has fewer calories and grams of fat than standard ground turkey, which can have as much as 15% fat. It also tastes fantastic and doesn't dry out when cooked. Just look for the kind labeled at least 96% fat-free or as having no more than 4% fat.

Prefer turkey? I've got you covered. Lean ground turkey (about 7% fat) is my number-one recommendation. It has a bit more calories and fat than extra-lean beef, but it's juicy, delicious, and all-around great. If you want nutritional stats closer to the extra-lean ground beef, reach for extra-lean ground turkey, which is typically labeled as 99% fat-free. It's not quite as flavorful, but it's still a solid pick!

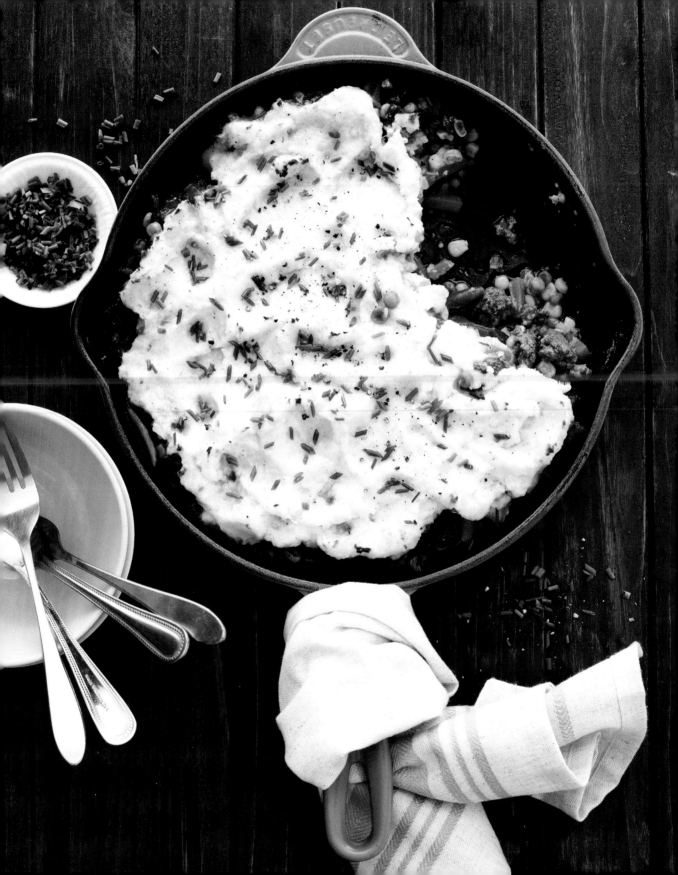

SIMPLE SHEPHERD'S PIE

¼th of recipe: 363 calories, 8.5g total fat (4g sat fat), 659mg sodium, 38g carbs, 6g fiber, 8g sugars, 31.5g protein

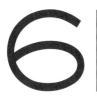

12 ounces (about 1 medium) **russet potato**
3 cups **cauliflower florets**
4 cups **frozen petite mixed vegetables**
1 cup **beef gravy**
1 pound **raw extra-lean ground beef**
¼ cup **light/reduced-fat cream cheese**

seasonings:
1 tablespoon dried minced onion
¼ teaspoon each salt and black pepper
1 teaspoon garlic powder

363 CALORIES

You'll need: medium pot, large microwave-safe bowl, large oven-safe skillet, nonstick spray, large bowl, potato masher

Prep: 10 minutes
Cook: 1 hour 5 minutes

EXTRA, EXTRA!

Chopped chives on top take this comfort food to the next level . . .

1. Preheat oven to 375 degrees.

2. Bring a medium pot of water to a boil. Peel and cube potato.

3. Add potato and cauliflower to the pot. Once returned to a boil, reduce heat to medium. Cook until very tender, 15 to 20 minutes.

4. Meanwhile, prepare mixed veggies and beef. Place mixed veggies in a large microwave-safe bowl. Cover and microwave for 3 minutes.

5. Stir mixed veggies, re-cover, and microwave for 1 more minute, or until thawed.

6. Drain excess water from mixed veggies. Add gravy, and stir to coat.

7. Bring a large oven-safe skillet sprayed with nonstick spray to medium-high heat on the stove. Add beef, and sprinkle with dried minced onion, salt, and ⅛ teaspoon pepper. Cook and crumble for about 5 minutes, until beef is fully cooked.

8. Evenly top with gravy-coated veggies, and remove from heat.

9. Drain cauliflower and potato, and transfer to a large bowl. Add cream cheese, garlic powder, and remaining ⅛ teaspoon pepper. Thoroughly mash and mix.

10. Evenly spoon into the skillet, and smooth out the top. Bake until filling is bubbly and top has slightly browned, about 35 minutes.

MAKES 4 SERVINGS

MEXI-LICIOUS ZUCCHINI BOATS

 ½ of recipe (2 stuffed zucchini halves): 303 calories, 11.5g total fat (5.5g sat fat), 461mg sodium, 16.5g carbs, 3.5g fiber, 8.5g sugars, 35g protein

2 medium-large **zucchini** (about 10 ounces each)
8 ounces **raw extra-lean ground beef**
¼ cup **frozen sweet corn kernels**
½ cup shredded **reduced-fat Mexican-blend cheese**
½ cup chopped **tomatoes**
¼ cup chopped **scallions**

seasonings:
2 teaspoons taco seasoning

You'll need: baking sheet, nonstick spray, skillet

Prep: 10 minutes
Cook: 10 minutes
Cool: 5 minutes

1. Preheat oven to broil. Spray a baking sheet with nonstick spray.

2. Pierce zucchini several times with a fork. Microwave for 3 minutes.

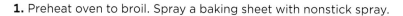

3. Flip zucchini and microwave for 3 more minutes, or until softened. Pat dry and let cool, about 5 minutes.

4. Meanwhile, bring a skillet sprayed with nonstick spray to medium-high heat. Add beef and 1½ teaspoons seasoning. Cook and crumble for about 4 minutes. Add corn. Cook and stir until corn has thawed and beef is fully cooked, about 1 minute.

5. Cut zucchini in half lengthwise. Gently scoop out and discard the inside flesh (or save for another time), leaving about ¼ inch inside the skin. Thoroughly pat dry. Sprinkle with remaining ½ teaspoon seasoning.

6. Place hollow zucchini halves on the baking sheet. Fill with beef mixture, and sprinkle with cheese.

7. Bake until zucchini is hot and cheese has melted, about 1 minute.

8. Top with tomatoes and scallions.

MAKES 2 SERVINGS

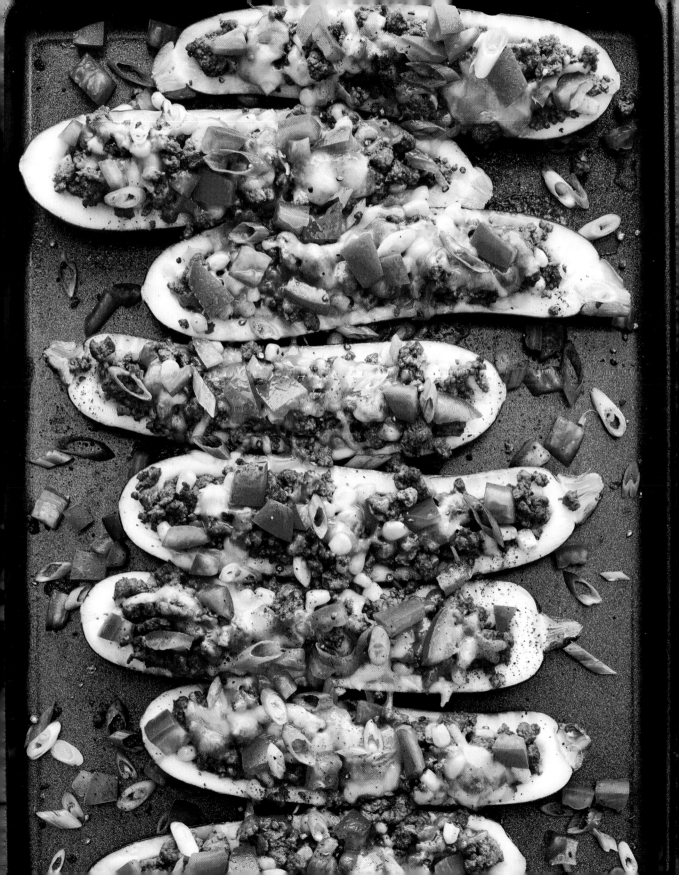

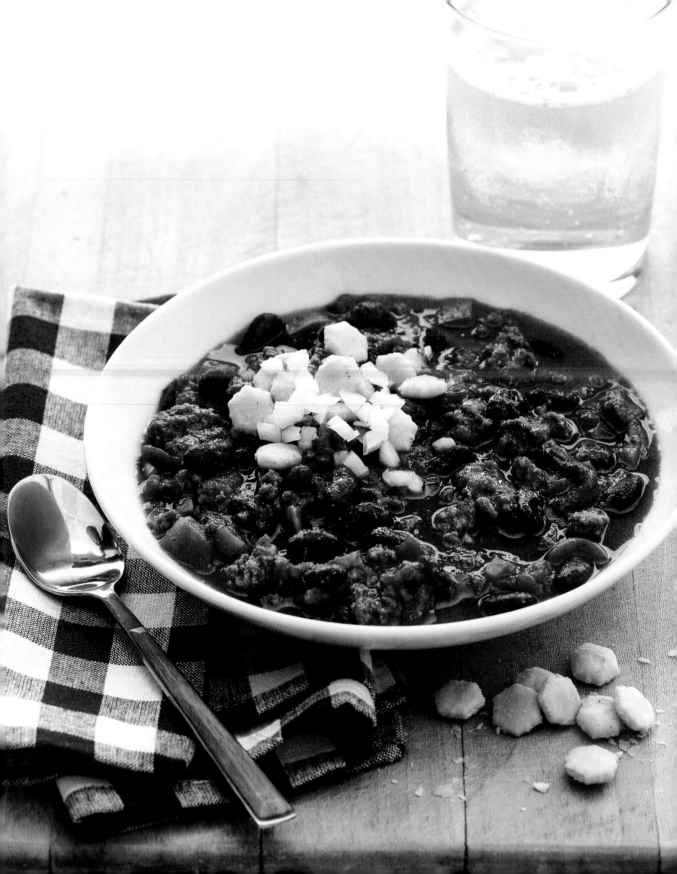

INSTANT-POT BEEF CHILI

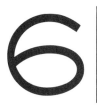 **⅙th of recipe (about 1 cup):** 214 calories, 3.5g total fat (1.5g sat fat), 741mg sodium, 23g carbs, 7g fiber, 7.5g sugars, 22g protein

6

1 pound **raw extra-lean ground beef**
One 15-ounce can **red kidney beans**, drained and rinsed
One 14.5-ounce can **crushed tomatoes**
One 14.5-ounce can **diced tomatoes with green chiles** (not drained)
1 cup chopped **onion**, or more for topping
1 cup chopped **bell pepper**

seasonings:
¼ teaspoon each salt and black pepper
1 tablespoon chili seasoning

214 CALORIES

You'll need: Instant Pot, nonstick spray

Prep: 5 minutes
Cook: 35 minutes
Cool: 10 minutes

1. Spray an Instant Pot with nonstick spray. Press Sauté, and add beef, salt, and black pepper. Cook and crumble until browned and mostly cooked, about 5 minutes.

2. Press Keep Warm/Cancel. Add remaining ingredients and seasoning, and mix well.

3. Seal with lid. Press Manual, and set for 10 minutes.

4. Once cooked, let sit for 10 minutes.

5. Press Keep Warm/Cancel. Vent to release steam.

MAKES 6 SERVINGS

EXTRA, EXTRA!

Oyster crackers are the perfect topping.

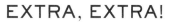

INSTANT-POT ITALIAN MEATBALLS

⅕th of recipe (4 meatballs with sauce): 213 calories, 6g total fat (2g sat fat), 559mg sodium, 15g carbs, 2.5g fiber, 7.5g sugars, 24g protein

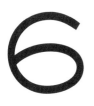

2 cups **marinara sauce** with 3g fat or less per serving
1 pound **raw extra-lean ground beef**
1 cup finely chopped **onion**
⅓ cup (about 2 large) **egg whites** or **fat-free liquid egg substitute**
¼ cup **whole-wheat panko breadcrumbs**
1 tablespoon grated **Parmesan cheese**, or more for topping

seasonings:
½ teaspoon Italian seasoning
½ teaspoon garlic powder
¼ teaspoon each salt and black pepper

213 CALORIES

You'll need: Instant Pot, nonstick spray, large bowl

Prep: 20 minutes
Cook: 25 minutes
Cool: 10 minutes

1. Add marinara sauce to an Instant Pot sprayed with nonstick spray.

2. In a large bowl, combine remaining ingredients and seasonings. Thoroughly mix.

3. Firmly and evenly form into 20 meatballs, and place in the pot.

4. Seal with lid. Press Manual, and set for 8 minutes.

5. Once cooked, press Keep Warm/Cancel. Let sit for 10 minutes.

6. Vent to release steam.

MAKES 5 SERVINGS

EXTRA, EXTRA!

Some like it hot . . . Try a sprinkle of red pepper flakes on your meatballs!

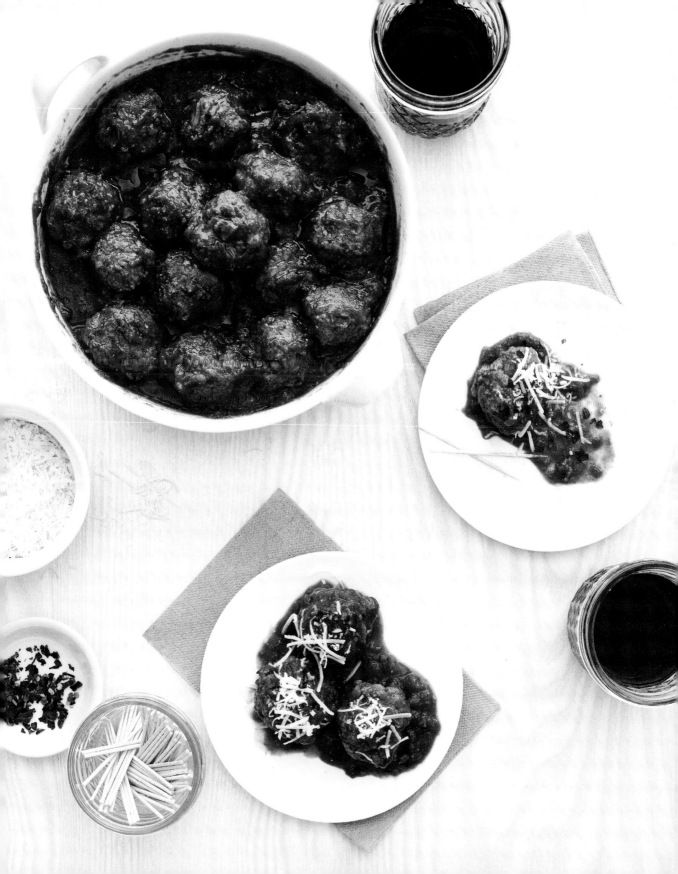

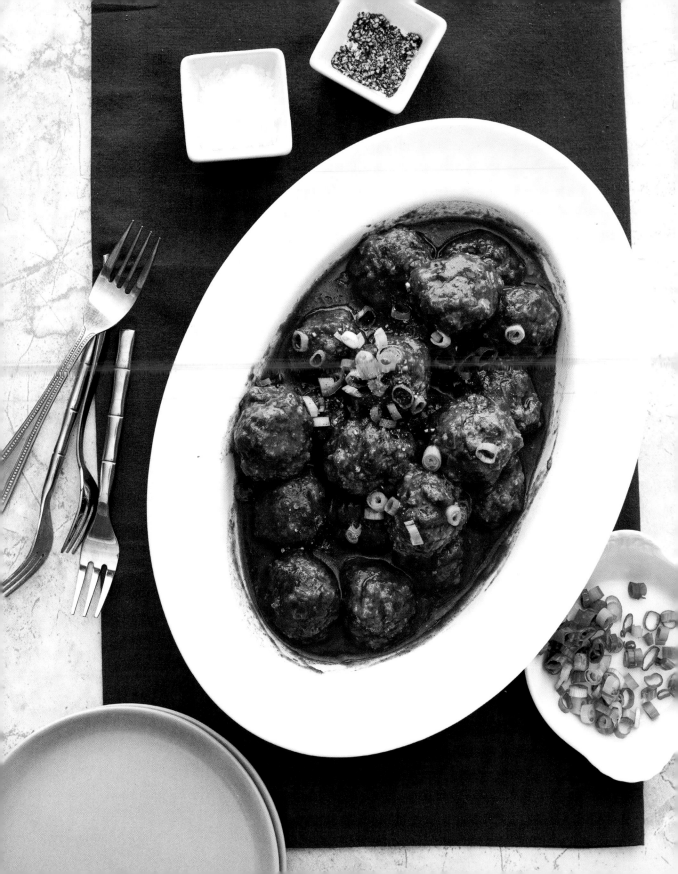

INSTANT-POT HONEY BBQ MEATBALLS

⅕th of recipe (4 meatballs with sauce): 258 calories, 4g total fat (1.5g sat fat), 629mg sodium, 33g carbs, 1g fiber, 25g sugars, 21.5g protein

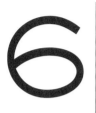

¾ cup **BBQ sauce** with 45 calories or less per 2-tablespoon serving
¼ cup **honey**
1 pound **raw extra-lean ground beef**
1 cup finely chopped **red onion**
⅓ cup (about 3 large) **egg whites** or **fat-free liquid egg substitute**
¼ cup **whole-wheat panko breadcrumbs**

seasonings:
½ teaspoon garlic powder
½ teaspoon onion powder
¼ teaspoon each salt and black pepper

258 CALORIES

You'll need: Instant Pot, nonstick spray, large bowl

Prep: 20 minutes
Cook: 20 minutes
Cool: 10 minutes

1. Spray an Instant Pot with nonstick spray. Add BBQ sauce, honey, and ¼ cup water. Stir until uniform.

2. In a large bowl, combine beef, onion, egg, breadcrumbs, and seasonings. Thoroughly mix.

3. Firmly and evenly form into 20 meatballs, and place in the pot.

4. Top with lid and seal. Press Manual, and set for 8 minutes.

5. Once cooked, press Keep Warm/Cancel. Let sit for 10 minutes.

6. Vent to release steam.

MAKES 5 SERVINGS

EXTRA, EXTRA!

Top with chopped scallions for a flavorful crunch and some color . . .

INSTANT-POT SLOPPY JANES

GF **⅕th of recipe (about ¾ cup):** 162 calories, 4g total fat (1.5g sat fat), 409mg sodium, 10g carbs, 1.5g fiber, 6g sugars, 20g protein

1 cup chopped **onion**
1 cup **canned crushed tomatoes**
1½ tablespoons **brown sugar** (not packed)
1 tablespoon **Worcestershire sauce**
1 tablespoon **red wine vinegar**
1 pound **raw extra-lean ground beef**

seasonings:
1 teaspoon garlic powder
1 teaspoon chili powder
½ teaspoon salt

You'll need:
Instant Pot

Prep: 10 minutes
Cook: 20 minutes
Cool: 10 minutes

1. In an Instant Pot, combine onion, crushed tomatoes, sugar, sauce, and vinegar. Stir until uniform.

2. Add beef and seasonings, and thoroughly mix.

3. Seal with lid. Press Manual, and set for 8 minutes.

4. Once cooked, press Keep Warm/Cancel. Let sit for 10 minutes.

5. Vent to release steam.

MAKES 5 SERVINGS

EXTRA, EXTRA!

Pile some onto a whole-grain roll, and top with pickles. Lunch is served!

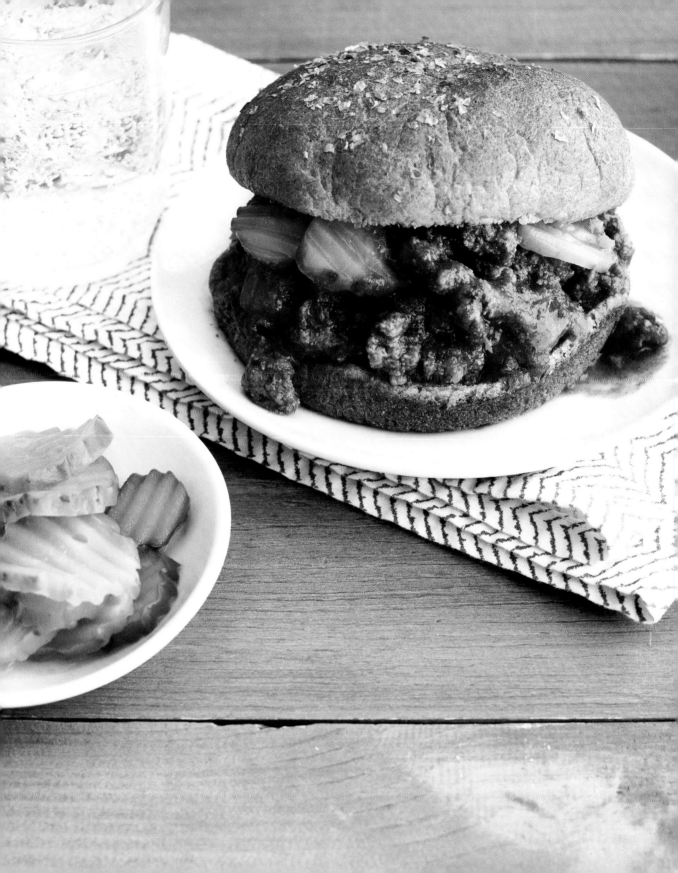

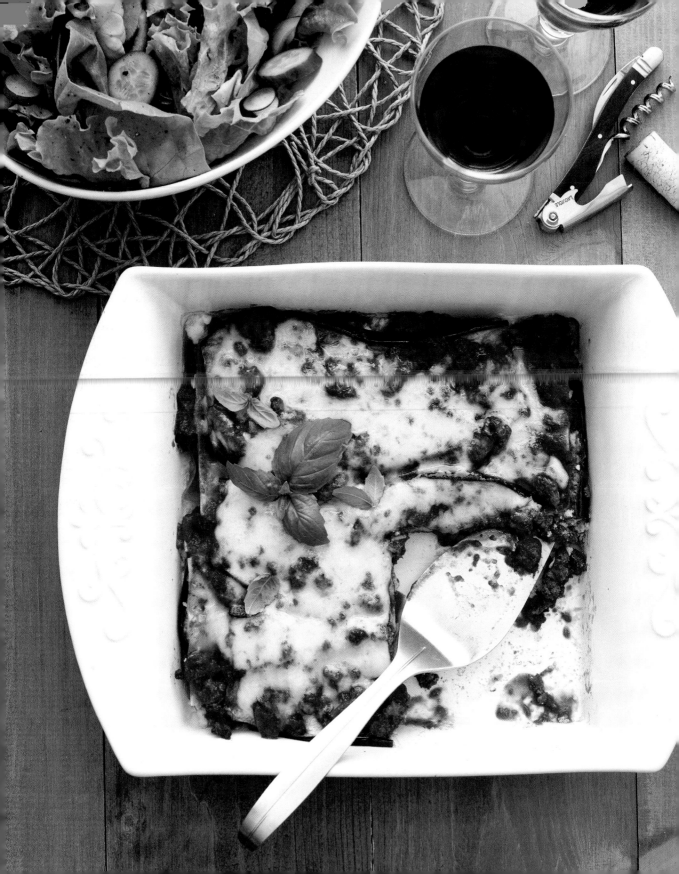

EGGPLANT LASAGNA

¼th of lasagna: 307 calories, 9g total fat (4.5g sat fat), 562mg sodium, 31.5g carbs, 7.5g fiber, 12.5g sugars, 26.5g protein

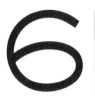

1 large **eggplant** (about 20 ounces), ends removed
8 ounces **raw extra-lean ground beef**
1 cup **marinara sauce** with 3g fat or less per serving
1 cup **light/low-fat ricotta cheese**
4 **whole-grain oven-ready lasagna sheets**
½ cup shredded **part-skim mozzarella cheese**

seasonings:
1 teaspoon garlic powder
¾ teaspoon onion powder
½ teaspoon Italian seasoning
¼ teaspoon each salt and black pepper

307 CALORIES

You'll need: baking sheet, 8-inch by 8-inch baking pan, nonstick spray, large skillet, medium bowl, foil

Prep: 20 minutes
Cook: 1 hour
Cool: 10 minutes

HG FYI

If needed, break lasagna sheets to fit the baking pan.

1. Preheat oven to 400 degrees. Spray a baking sheet and an 8-inch by 8-inch baking pan with nonstick spray.

2. Cut eggplant lengthwise into ½-inch slices. Sprinkle with ½ teaspoon each garlic powder and onion powder.

3. Place on the baking sheet, and bake for 10 minutes.

4. Meanwhile, bring a large skillet sprayed with nonstick spray to medium-high heat. Add beef, Italian seasoning, ¼ teaspoon garlic powder, salt, pepper, and remaining ¼ teaspoon onion powder. Cook and crumble for about 5 minutes, until fully cooked. Remove from heat, and mix in marinara sauce.

5. Flip eggplant. Bake until lightly browned and softened, about 10 minutes.

6. In a medium bowl, mix ricotta with remaining ¼ teaspoon garlic powder.

7. Blot eggplant dry. In the baking pan, evenly layer ⅓rd of the eggplant, half of the seasoned ricotta, 2 lasagna sheets, and ⅓rd of the meat sauce.

8. Repeat layering. Evenly top with remaining eggplant and meat sauce.

9. Top with mozzarella. Cover with foil, and bake for 30 minutes.

10. Uncover and bake until lasagna sheets are cooked through and cheese has lightly browned, about 8 minutes.

11. Let cool for 10 minutes before slicing.

MAKES 4 SERVINGS

SAUCY STUFFED PEPPERS

GF **¼th of recipe (1 stuffed pepper):** 292 calories, 8g total fat (3g sat fat), 589mg sodium, 25.5g carbs, 7g fiber, 14g sugars, 30.5g protein

6

4 large **bell peppers** (look for ones that sit flat)
1 pound **raw extra-lean ground beef**
2 cups **riced cauliflower**
1 cup chopped **onion**
1½ cups **marinara sauce** with 3g fat or less per serving
¼ cup shredded **part-skim mozzarella cheese**

seasonings:
1 teaspoon garlic powder
1 teaspoon onion powder
¾ teaspoon Italian seasoning
¼ teaspoon each salt and black pepper

292 CALORIES

You'll need: 8-inch by 8-inch baking pan, large skillet, nonstick spray

Prep: 15 minutes
Cook: 35 minutes

1. Preheat oven to 400 degrees.

2. Slice off and discard stem ends of bell peppers. Remove and discard seeds.

3. Place peppers in an 8-inch by 8-inch baking pan, cut sides up. Bake until soft, 25 to 30 minutes. Meanwhile, prepare filling.

4. Bring a large skillet sprayed with nonstick spray to medium-high heat. Add beef, cauliflower, onion, and seasonings. Cook and stir for 8 to 10 minutes, until beef has fully cooked and veggies have softened.

5. Reduce skillet heat to low, and add sauce. Cook and stir until hot, about 2 minutes.

6. Blot away excess moisture from bell peppers. Evenly fill, and sprinkle with cheese.

7. Bake until cheese melts, about 5 minutes.

MAKES 4 SERVINGS

HG FYI

Don't miss the cauliflower rice guide on page 365 . . .

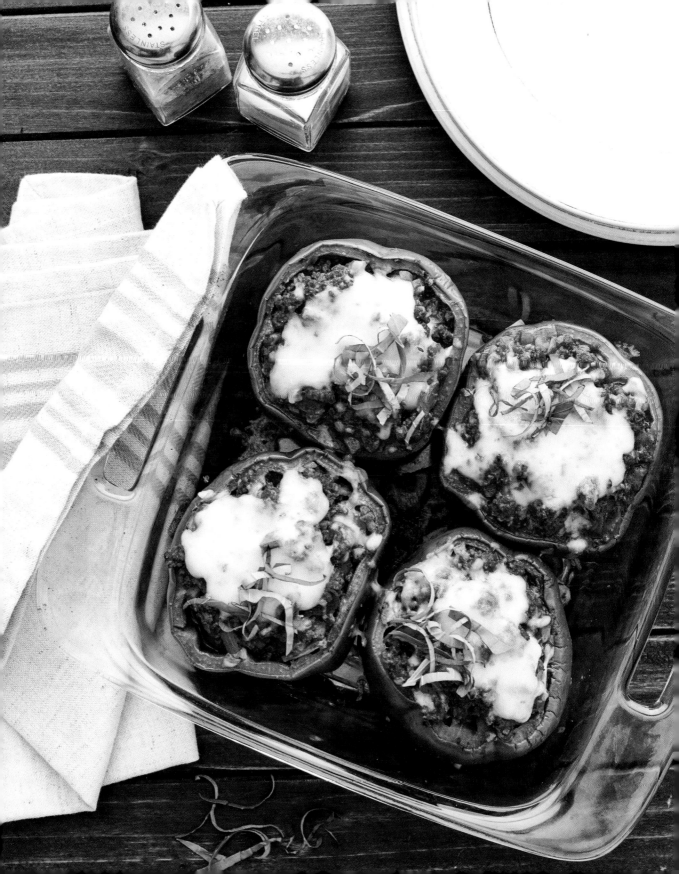

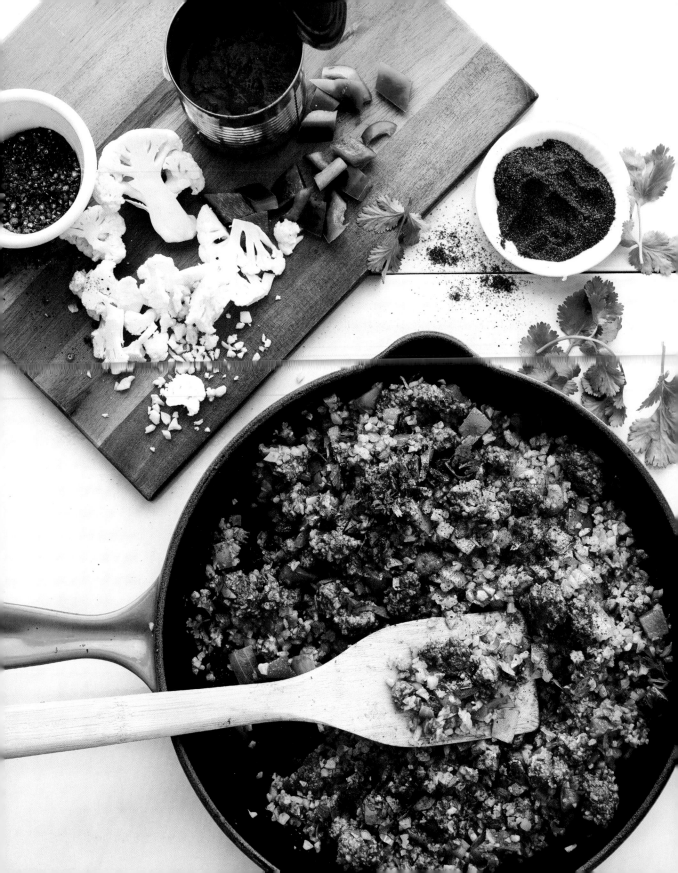

BEEFY CAULIFLOWER RICE STIR-FRY

 GF **½ of recipe (about 2¼ cups):** 292 calories, 5.5g total fat (2.5g sat fat), 656mg sodium, 30g carbs, 9.5g fiber, 12g sugars, 32g protein

6

1 cup **canned crushed tomatoes**
8 ounces **raw extra-lean ground beef**
½ cup chopped **green bell pepper**
½ cup chopped **onion**
1 tablespoon chopped **garlic**
4 cups **riced cauliflower**

seasonings:
1½ teaspoons taco seasoning
⅛ teaspoon each salt and black pepper

292 CALORIES

You'll need: medium bowl, large skillet with lid, nonstick spray

Prep: 5 minutes
Cook: 15 minutes

1. In a medium bowl, mix crushed tomatoes with 1 teaspoon taco seasoning.

2. Bring a large skillet sprayed with nonstick spray to medium-high heat. Add beef, and sprinkle with salt, black pepper, and remaining ½ teaspoon taco seasoning. Add bell pepper, onion, and garlic. Cook and crumble until beef has browned and veggies have slightly softened, about 4 minutes.

3. Mix in cauliflower. Cover and cook for 3 minutes.

4. Remove lid, and cook and stir until beef is fully cooked and cauliflower is tender, about 3 more minutes.

5. Reduce heat to low. Add seasoned tomatoes. Cook and stir until hot, about 2 minutes.

MAKES 2 SERVINGS

HG FYI

Flip to page 365 for Cauliflower Rice Made Simple!

JUMBO BURGER PATTIES

¼th of recipe (1 patty): 193 calories, 5g total fat (2g sat fat), 381mg sodium, 8.5g carbs, 1g fiber, 3g sugars, 26.5g protein

1 pound **raw extra-lean ground beef**
1½ cups finely chopped **mushrooms**
⅓ cup **whole-wheat panko breadcrumbs**
¼ cup (about 2 large) **egg whites** or **fat-free liquid egg substitute**
2 tablespoons **ketchup**
1 tablespoon **yellow mustard**

seasonings:
½ teaspoon garlic powder
¼ teaspoon each salt and black pepper

193 CALORIES

You'll need: large bowl, grill pan (or extra-large skillet), nonstick spray

Prep: 15 minutes
Cook: 25 minutes

1. Place ingredients and seasonings in a large bowl. Thoroughly mix.

2. Evenly form into 4 patties, about ¾ inch thick.

3. Bring a grill pan (or extra-large skillet) sprayed with nonstick spray to medium-high heat. In batches of 2, cook patties for about 6 minutes per side, until cooked to your preference. (Reduce cook time for rare; increase for well done.)

MAKES 4 SERVINGS

HUNGRY FOR MORE?

Don't miss the Butternut Veggie Burgers on page 229!

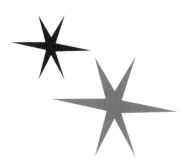

6 Staples for Your Burger Spread

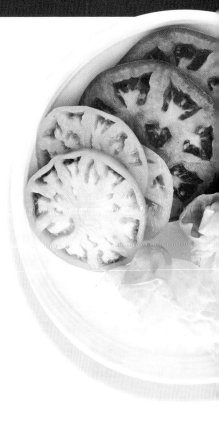

1. **Whole-grain buns.** Look for ones with 150 calories or less. I LOVE flat sandwich buns and light English muffins!

2. **Pickles.** Serve spears on the side, or pile pickle chips on top of your burger patty.

3. **Onion.** Red, white, sliced, chopped . . . You can't go wrong!

4. **Lettuce.** Big leaves are perfect for burger topping OR bun replacing! Protein-style burger, anyone?

5. **Tomato.** Choose classic red or vibrant yellow . . . Romas are my favorite.

6. **Ketchup & mustard.** The ultimate condiment couple gets paired up on this list. Mix 'em together for a special sauce!

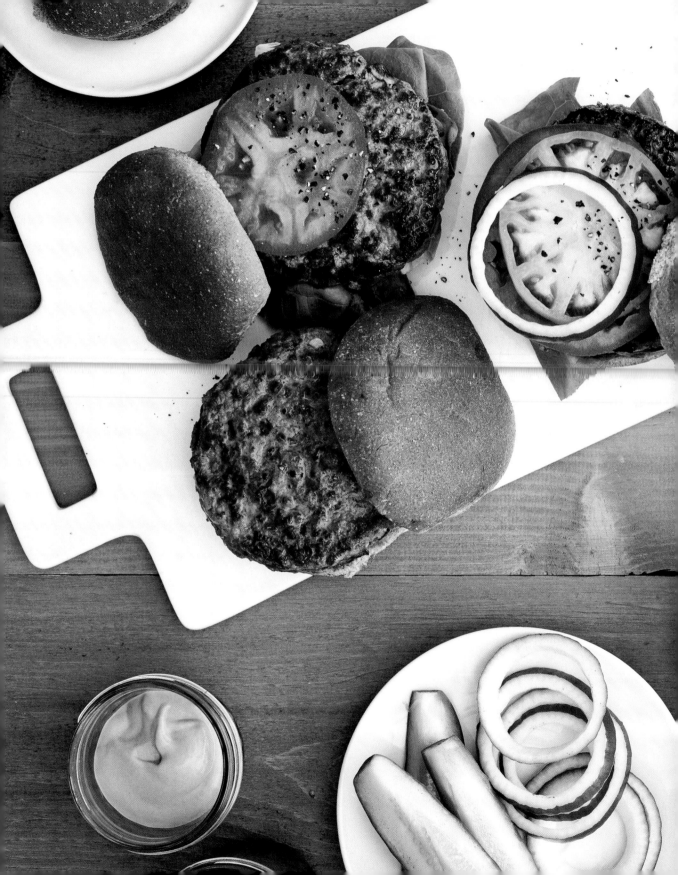

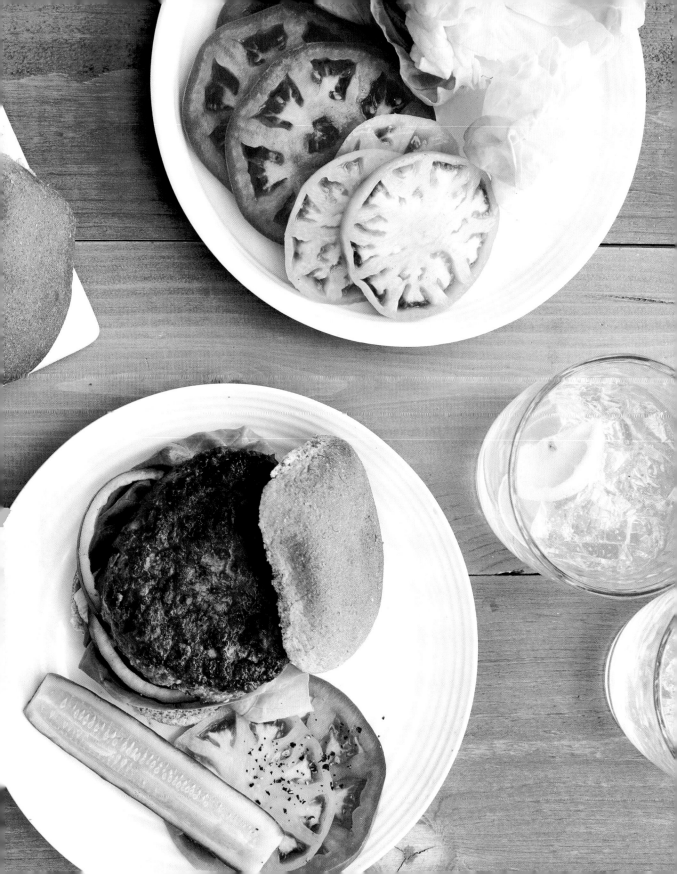

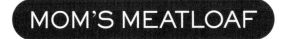

MOM'S MEATLOAF

⅕th of meatloaf: 187 calories, 4g total fat (1.5g sat fat), 476mg sodium, 13g carbs, 1.5g fiber, 5g sugars, 23.5g protein

1 pound **raw extra-lean ground beef**
1½ cups finely chopped **brown mushrooms**
¾ cup finely chopped **onion**
½ cup (about 4 large) **egg whites** or **fat-free liquid egg substitute**
½ cup **whole-wheat panko breadcrumbs**
¼ cup **ketchup**

seasonings:
2 teaspoons garlic powder
½ teaspoon salt
¼ teaspoon black pepper

187 CALORIES

You'll need: 9-inch by 5-inch loaf pan, nonstick spray, large bowl

Prep: 20 minutes
Cook: 50 minutes
Cool: 10 minutes

1. Preheat oven to 350 degrees. Spray a 9-inch by 5-inch loaf pan with nonstick spray.

2. In a large bowl, combine beef, mushrooms, onion, egg, breadcrumbs, and seasonings. Mix thoroughly.

3. Transfer to the baking pan, and smooth out the top.

4. Spread with ketchup. Bake until cooked through, about 50 minutes.

5. Let set for 10 minutes before slicing.

MAKES 5 SERVINGS

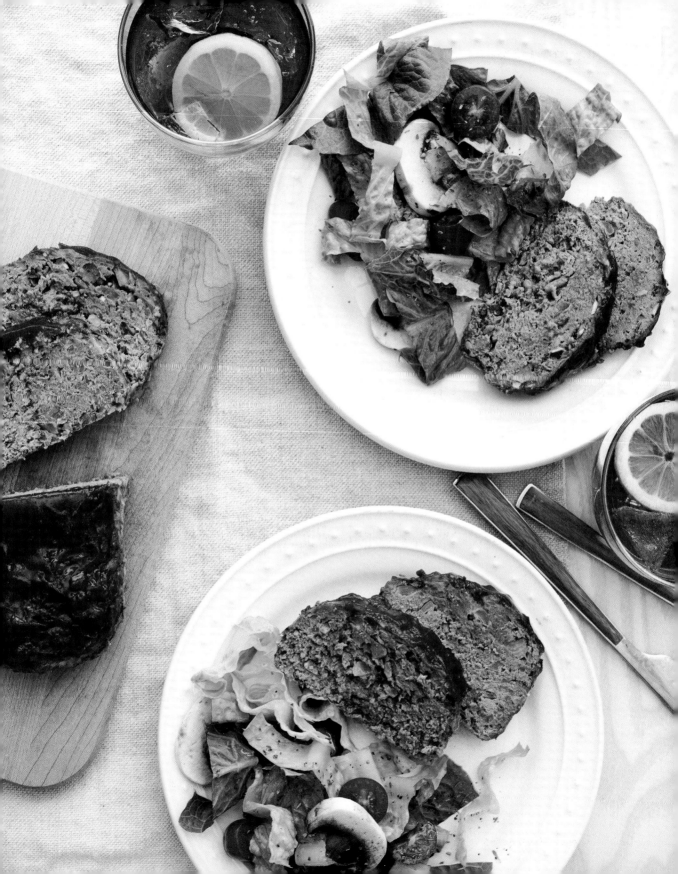

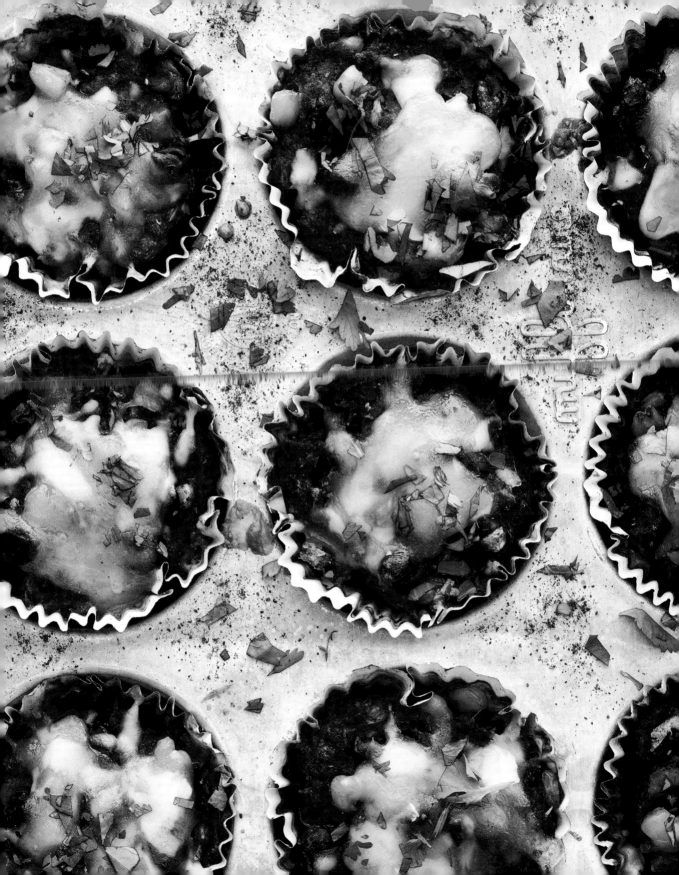

TEX-MEX MEATLOAF MINIS

⅛th of recipe (2 meatloaf minis): 189 calories, 5.5g total fat (2.5g sat fat), 314mg sodium, 13g carbs, 2.5g fiber, 2g sugars, 20g protein

1 pound **raw extra-lean ground beef**
¾ cup **canned crushed tomatoes**
½ cup **whole-wheat panko breadcrumbs**
½ cup **canned black beans**, drained and rinsed
½ cup **frozen sweet corn kernels**
½ cup shredded **reduced-fat Mexican-blend cheese**

seasonings:
1 tablespoon taco seasoning

You'll need: 12-cup muffin pan, foil baking cups (or nonstick spray), large bowl

Prep: 15 minutes
Cook: 40 minutes

1. Preheat oven to 350 degrees. Line a 12-cup muffin pan with foil baking cups, or spray it with nonstick spray.

2. In a large bowl, combine beef, tomatoes, breadcrumbs, beans, corn, and seasoning. Mix thoroughly.

3. Evenly fill muffin pan, and smooth out the tops. Bake until firm and cooked through with lightly browned edges, about 35 minutes.

4. Top with cheese. Bake until melted, about 3 minutes.

MAKES 6 SERVINGS

ASIAN-STYLE MINI MEATLOAVES

⅙th of recipe (2 mini meatloaves): 151 calories, 3.5g total fat (1.5g sat fat), 358mg sodium, 10g carbs, 1.5g fiber, 4g sugars, 18g protein

2 cups **frozen Asian-style stir-fry vegetables**
1 pound **raw extra-lean ground beef**
½ cup **whole-wheat panko breadcrumbs**
¼ cup (about 2 large) **egg whites** or **fat-free liquid egg substitute**
2 tablespoons **sweet Asian chili sauce**, or more for topping

seasonings:
½ teaspoon garlic powder
½ teaspoon onion powder
½ teaspoon salt

You'll need: 12-cup muffin pan, foil baking cups (or nonstick spray), large microwave-safe bowl

Prep: 10 minutes
Cook: 35 minutes

1. Preheat oven to 375 degrees. Line a 12-cup muffin pan with foil baking cups, or spray it with nonstick spray.

2. Place frozen veggies in a large microwave-safe bowl. Cover and microwave for 2 minutes, or until thawed.

3. Drain water, and roughly chop veggies.

4. Return veggies to the large bowl. Add remaining ingredients and seasonings.

5. Evenly fill muffin pan, and smooth out the tops. Bake until firm with lightly browned edges, about 30 minutes.

MAKES 6 SERVINGS

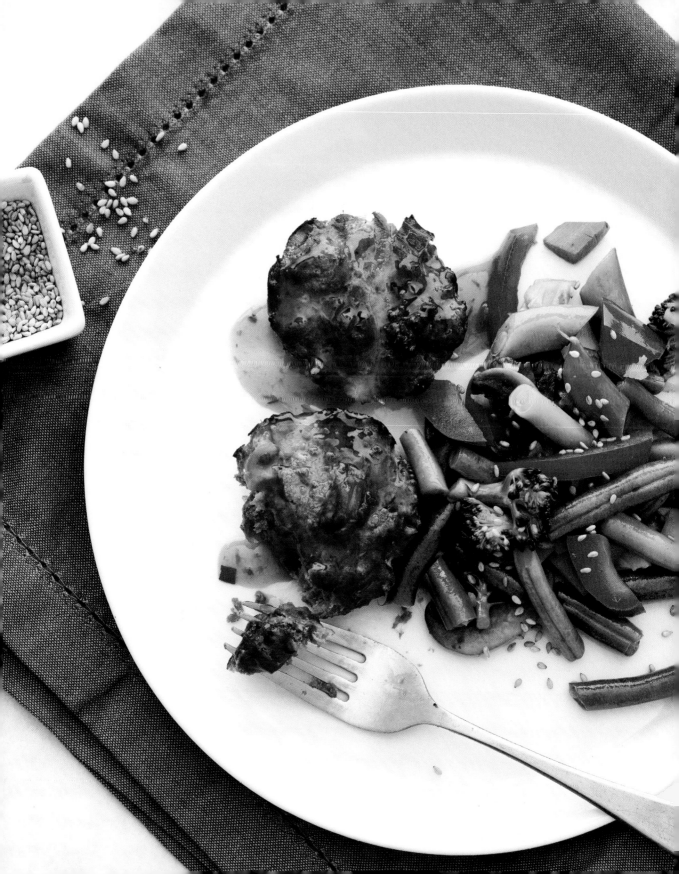

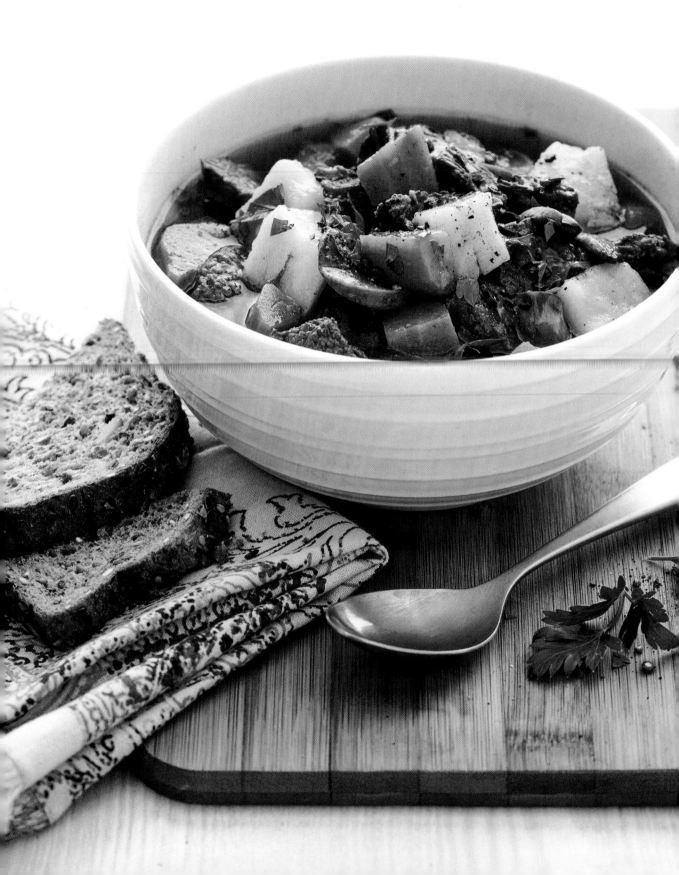

INSTANT-POT CHUNKY BEEF SOUP

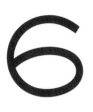 **⅙th of recipe (about 1½ cups):** 294 calories, 9.5g total fat (4g sat fat), 678mg sodium, 18g carbs, 3g fiber, 5.5g sugars, 35.5g protein

6

2 pounds **raw boneless beef chuck roast**, trimmed of excess fat, cut into bite-sized pieces
3 cups **reduced-sodium beef broth**
2½ cups chopped **carrots**
2 cups sliced **mushrooms**
1½ cups chopped **onion**
8 ounces (about 1 small-to-medium) **russet potato**, peeled and cubed

seasonings:
1 teaspoon garlic powder
¾ teaspoon salt
¼ teaspoon black pepper
¼ teaspoon ground thyme

You'll need: Instant Pot, nonstick spray

Prep: 25 minutes
Cook: 45 minutes
Cool: 10 minutes

1. Spray an Instant Pot with nonstick spray. Press Sauté, and add beef and seasonings. Cook and rotate until evenly browned, 6 to 8 minutes.

2. Press Keep Warm/Cancel. Add remaining ingredients, and mix well.

3. Seal with lid. Press Manual, and set for 20 minutes.

4. Press Keep Warm/Cancel. Let sit for 10 minutes.

5. Vent to release steam.

MAKES 6 SERVINGS

GO-TO GOULASH

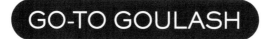

30m **½ of recipe (about 2 cups):** 283 calories, 8.5g total fat (3g sat fat), 661mg sodium, 22.5g carbs, 4.5g fiber, 11.5g sugars, 31g protein

1 pound (about 2 medium) **yellow squash**
8 ounces **raw lean flank steak**, thinly sliced
2 cups sliced **mushrooms**
1 cup chopped **onion**
½ cup **beef gravy**
1 tablespoon chopped **chives**

seasonings:
¼ teaspoon garlic powder
¼ teaspoon onion powder
¼ teaspoon salt
⅛ teaspoon black pepper
⅛ teaspoon ground thyme

283 CALORIES

You'll need: veggie peeler, large skillet, nonstick spray, strainer

Prep: 15 minutes
Cook: 15 minutes

1. Slice off and discard squash ends. Using a veggie peeler, slice squash into wide strips, rotating it after each slice.

2. Bring a large skillet sprayed with nonstick spray to medium-high heat. Cook and stir squash until slightly softened, about 4 minutes.

3. Transfer to a strainer, and thoroughly drain.

4. Remove skillet from heat, respray, and return to medium-high heat. Add steak, and sprinkle with seasonings. Add veggies, and cook and stir for about 4 minutes, until steak is fully cooked and veggies have softened.

5. Return squash to the skillet. Add gravy, and cook and stir until hot and well mixed, about 2 minutes.

6. Top with chives.

MAKES 2 SERVINGS

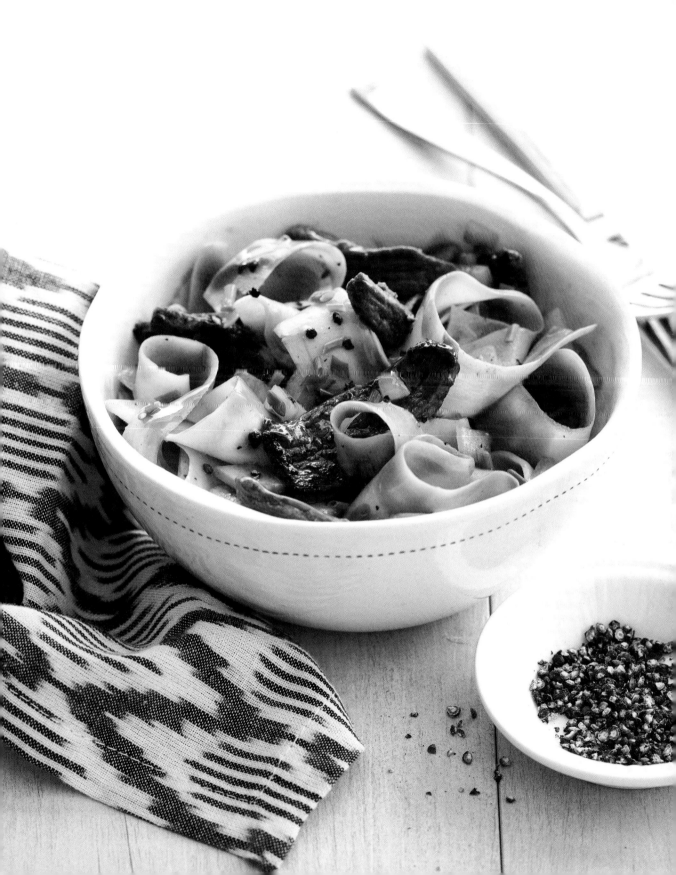

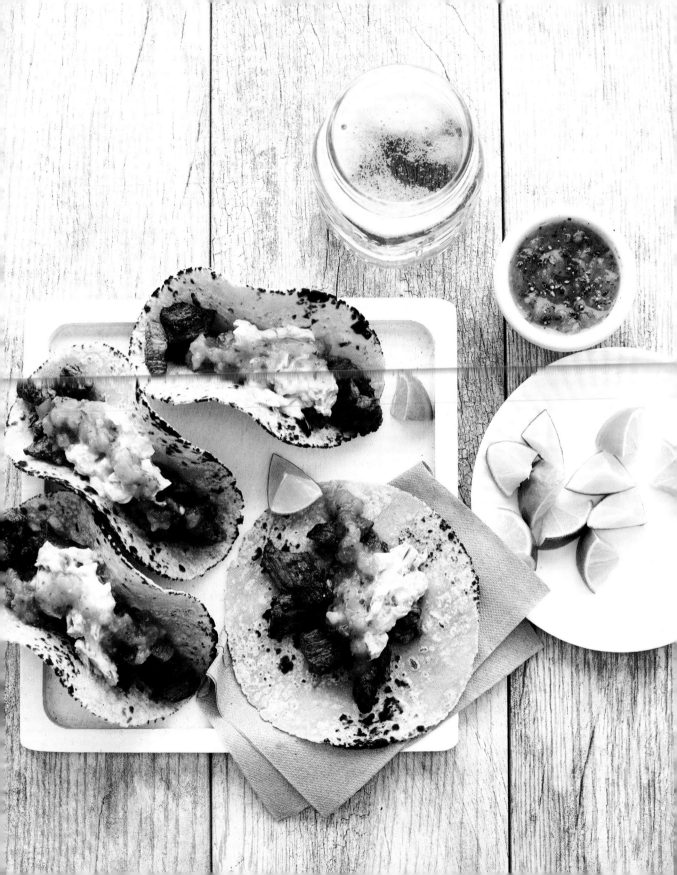

STEAK & AVOCADO SOFT TACOS

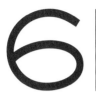

½ of recipe (2 tacos): 314 calories, 9.5g total fat (2.5g sat fat), 469mg sodium, 26g carbs, 3g fiber, 4g sugars, 30g protein

6

1½ teaspoons **lime juice**
8 ounces chopped **raw lean flank steak**
¼ cup **fat-free plain Greek yogurt**
1 ounce (about 2 tablespoons) mashed **avocado**
Four **6-inch corn tortillas**
¼ cup **salsa** (traditional or salsa verde)

seasonings:
½ teaspoon plus ⅛ teaspoon taco seasoning
⅛ teaspoon salt

You'll need: medium bowl, small bowl, large skillet, nonstick spray, paper towels

Prep: 10 minutes
Cook: 5 minutes

1. In a medium bowl, mix lime juice with ¼ teaspoon taco seasoning. Add steak, and stir to coat.

2. In a small bowl, combine yogurt, avocado, salt, and remaining ⅛ teaspoon taco seasoning. Mix until uniform.

3. Bring a large skillet sprayed with nonstick spray to medium-high heat. Cook and stir steak for about 4 minutes, until cooked through.

4. Place tortillas between 2 damp paper towels. Microwave for 20 seconds, or until warm and pliable.

5. Top tortillas with steak, avocado sauce, and salsa.

MAKES 2 SERVINGS

HG TIP

For extra flavor, char your tortillas in a dry skillet over high heat.

EASY-PEASY SLOW-COOKER PULLED PORK

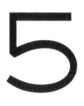

⅙th of recipe (about ¾ cup): 230 calories, 4.5g total fat (1.5g sat fat), 586mg sodium, 22g carbs, 1g fiber, 15.5g sugars, 23g protein

5

12 ounces **raw lean boneless pork tenderloin**, trimmed of excess fat

12 ounces **raw boneless pork shoulder** (the leanest piece you can find), trimmed of excess fat

2 cups roughly chopped **onion**

1 cup **BBQ sauce** with 45 calories or less per 2-tablespoon serving

½ cup **canned crushed pineapple packed in juice** (not drained)

seasonings:
⅛ teaspoon each salt and black pepper

230 CALORIES

You'll need: slow cooker, large bowl

Prep: 15 minutes
Cook: 3 to 4 hours or 7 to 8 hours

1. Place all the pork in a slow cooker, and season with salt and pepper. Add remaining ingredients, and lightly stir.

2. Cover and cook on high for 3 to 4 hours or on low for 7 to 8 hours, until pork is cooked through.

3. Transfer pork to a large bowl, and shred with two forks.

4. Return pork to the slow cooker, and mix well.

MAKES 6 SERVINGS

6 SIMPLE WAYS TO SERVE IT . . .

1. **On a light or whole-grain bun**
2. **Over baked chips with reduced-fat cheese**
3. **In tacos (hard or soft)**
4. **In crispy wonton cups (page 328)**
5. **Wrapped in steamed cabbage leaves**
6. **Over shredded lettuce**

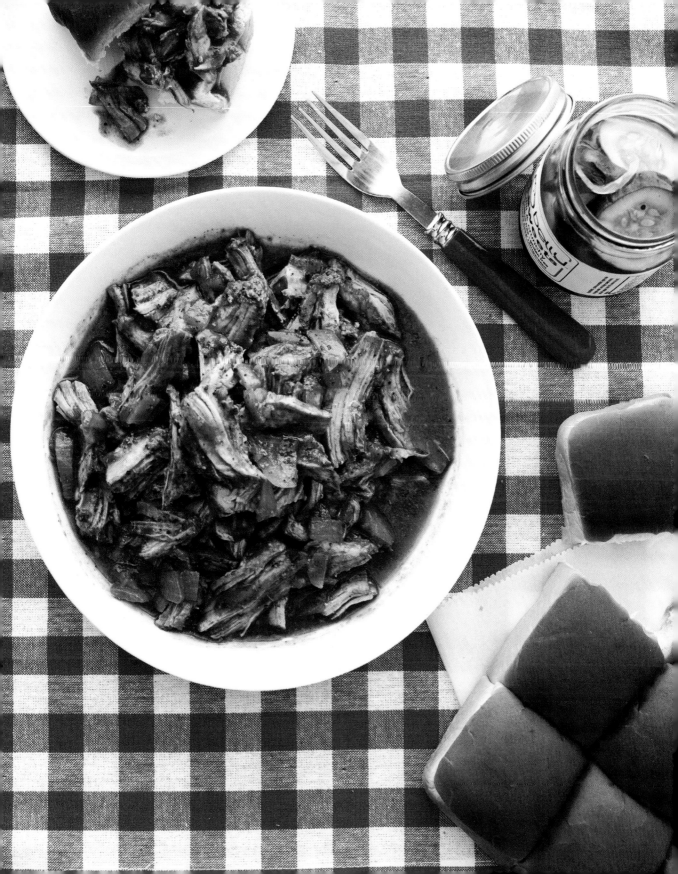

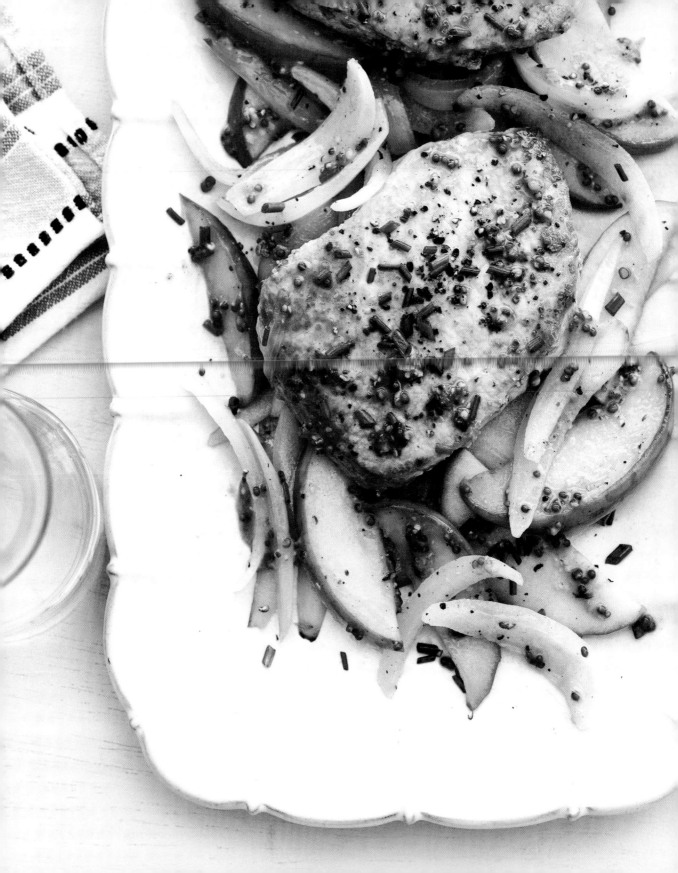

RETRO PORK CHOPS & APPLES

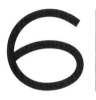 **½ of recipe:** 238 calories, 5g total fat (1.5g sat fat), 470mg sodium, 13.5g carbs, 2g fiber, 8.5g sugars, 33g protein

6

Two 5-ounce **boneless pork chops** trimmed of excess fat
1 cup (about 1 medium) sliced **apple**
1 cup (about 1 medium) sliced **onion**
1 tablespoon **brown or stone-ground mustard**
1 tablespoon **apple cider vinegar**
1 tablespoon chopped **chives**

seasonings:
¼ teaspoon each salt and black pepper

238 CALORIES

You'll need: large skillet, nonstick spray, plate

Prep: 10 minutes
Cook: 20 minutes

1. Bring a large skillet sprayed with nonstick spray to medium heat. Season pork chops with ⅛ teaspoon each salt and pepper. Cook for 3 minutes per side, or until cooked to your preference. Plate and cover to keep warm.

2. Remove skillet from heat; clean, if needed. Respray, and return to medium heat. Add apple, onion, and remaining ⅛ teaspoon each salt and pepper. Cook and stir until softened and lightly browned, 10 to 12 minutes.

3. Reduce heat to low. Add mustard and vinegar. Cook and stir until hot and well mixed, about 1 minute.

4. Serve topped with chives.

MAKES 2 SERVINGS

HULA CAULIFLOWER FRIED RICE

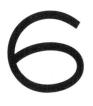 **¼th of recipe (about 1¼ cups):** 133 calories, 1g total fat (<0.5g sat fat), 677mg sodium, 21g carbs, 4g fiber, 12g sugars, 10.5g protein

6

½ cup (about 4 large) **egg whites** or **fat-free liquid egg substitute**
2 cups frozen **Asian-style stir-fry vegetables**
4 cups **riced cauliflower**
3 ounces (about 5 slices) **reduced-sodium ham**, chopped
½ cup **canned crushed pineapple packed in juice**, lightly drained
¼ cup **thick teriyaki sauce or marinade**

seasonings:
½ teaspoon garlic powder
⅛ teaspoon black pepper

You'll need: extra-large skillet (or wok) with lid, nonstick spray, bowl

Prep: 5 minutes
Cook: 20 minutes

1. Bring an extra-large skillet (or wok) sprayed with nonstick spray to medium heat.

2. Scramble egg until fully cooked, 3 to 4 minutes. Transfer to a bowl.

3. Remove skillet from heat; clean, if needed. Respray, and bring to medium-high heat. Add frozen veggies and 2 tablespoons water. Cover and cook for 2 minutes, or until thawed.

4. Add cauliflower and seasonings. Cook and stir until mostly softened, 6 to 8 minutes.

5. Reduce heat to medium low. Add scrambled egg, ham, pineapple, and teriyaki sauce. Cook and stir until hot and well mixed, about 2 minutes.

MAKES 4 SERVINGS

EXTRA, EXTRA!

Add chopped scallions for fresh flavor . . . Yum!

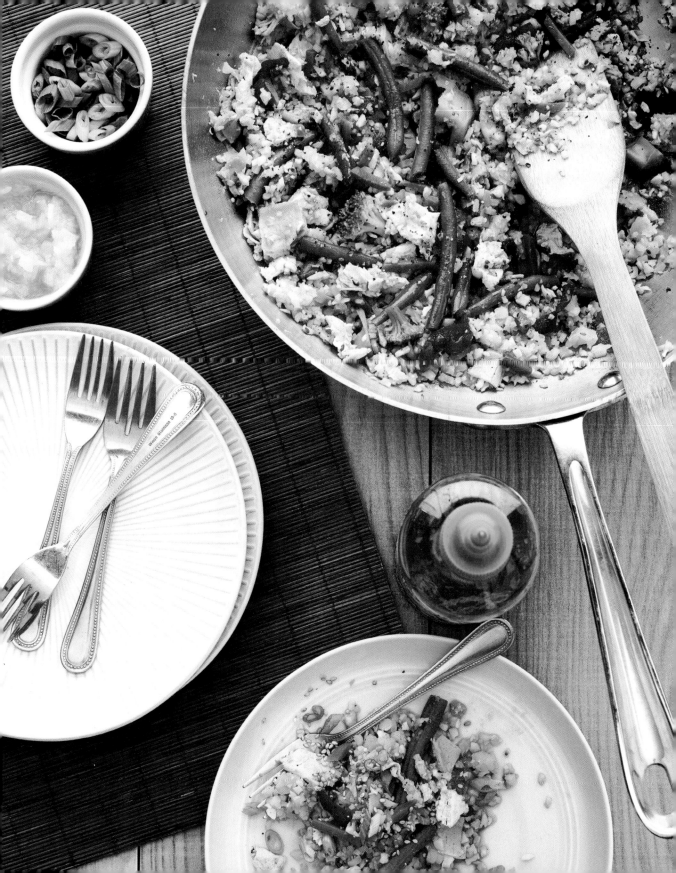

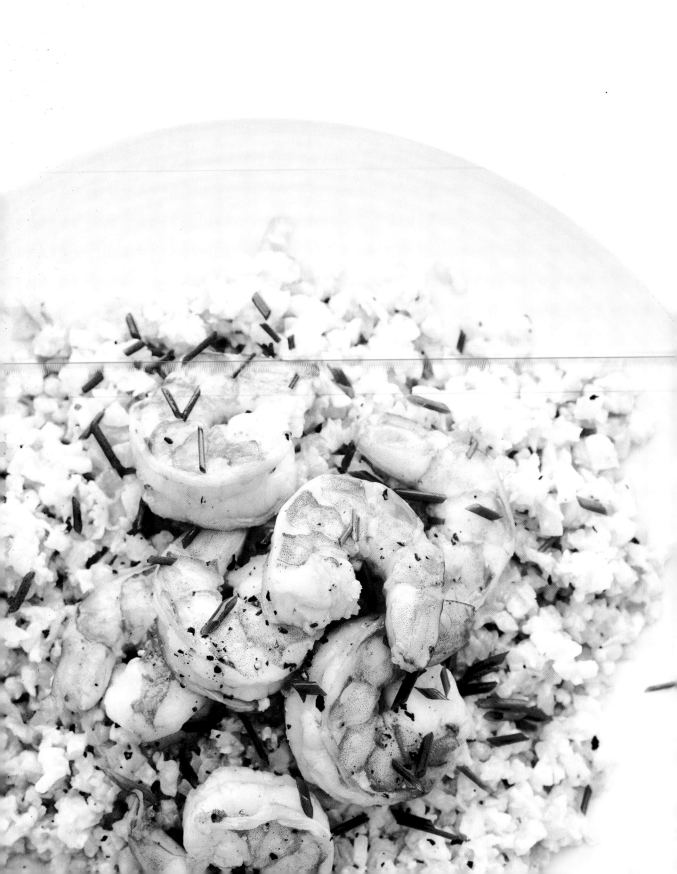

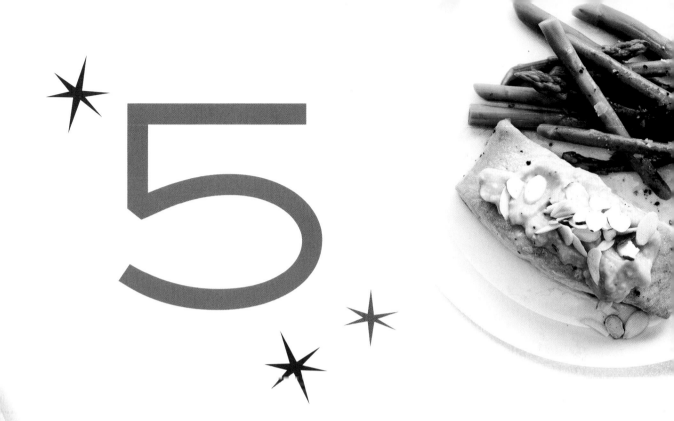

5

SIMPLY
SEAFOOD

You'll want to dive face first into these fish and shrimp dishes. And here's a smart shopping tip: Shop for seafood in the freezer aisle. It's generally cheaper than the stuff at the fish counter, which is often previously frozen anyway! And it'll last for quite a while in your freezer.

SHEET-PAN SHRIMP BAKE

30m **GF** **½ of recipe (about 2 cups):** 271 calories, 8.5g total fat (2.5g sat fat), 843mg sodium, 16.5g carbs, 3g fiber, 5g sugars, 32.5g protein

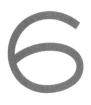

6 ounces (about 12) **raw large shrimp**, peeled, tails removed, deveined
2 teaspoons **lemon juice**
6 ounces (about 2 links) **fully cooked chicken sausage**, sliced into coins
1 cup **cherry tomatoes**, halved
½ cup **frozen sweet corn kernels**
3 cups roughly chopped **spinach**

seasonings:
½ teaspoon garlic powder
⅛ teaspoon black pepper
½ teaspoon Cajun seasoning

271 CALORIES

You'll need: baking sheet, nonstick spray, large bowl

Prep: 15 minutes
Cook: 15 minutes

1. Preheat oven to 400 degrees. Spray a baking sheet with nonstick spray.

2. In a large bowl, combine shrimp, lemon juice, garlic powder, and pepper. Toss to coat.

3. Add sausage, tomatoes, corn, and Cajun seasoning. Mix well.

4. Place spinach on the center of the baking sheet. Evenly top with contents of the bowl.

5. Bake until shrimp are cooked through and veggies have softened and lightly browned, about 12 minutes.

MAKES 2 SERVINGS

HG TIP

For added heat and flavor, stir in more Cajun seasoning . . .

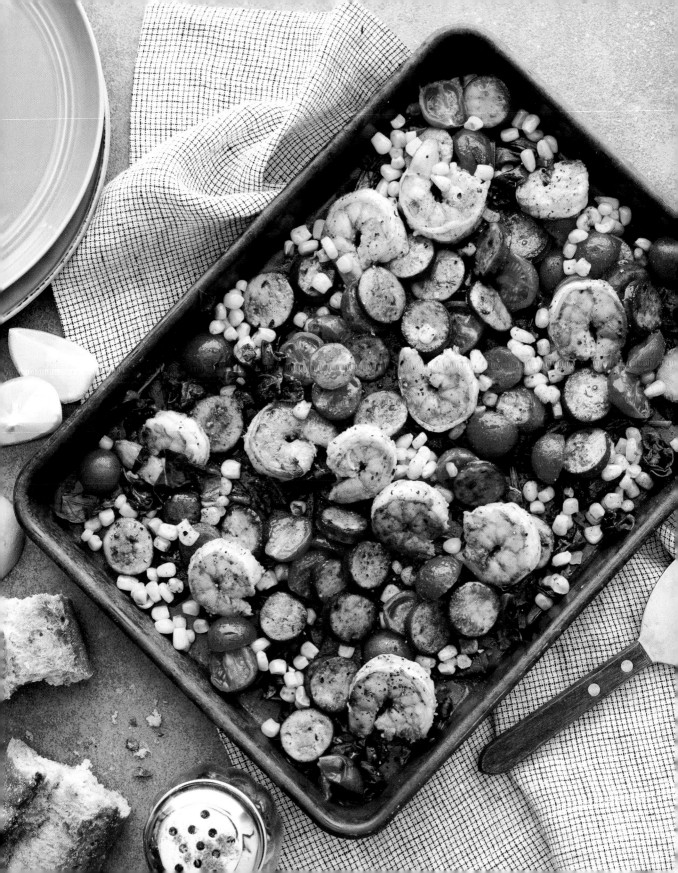

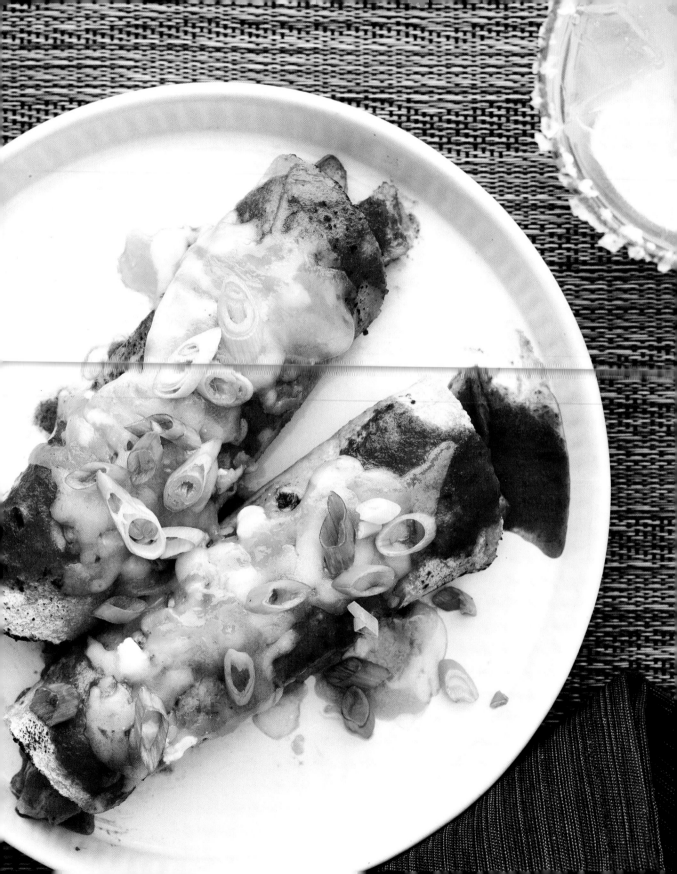

BLACKENED SHRIMP ENCHILADAS

GF **½ of recipe (2 enchiladas):** 293 calories, 9.5g total fat (4g sat fat), 796mg sodium, 27g carbs, 2.5g fiber, 2.5g sugars, 24.5g protein

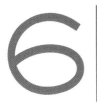

2 tablespoons **light/reduced-fat cream cheese**
½ cup **red enchilada sauce**
6 ounces (about 12) **raw large shrimp**, peeled, tails
    removed, deveined
Four **6-inch corn tortillas**
⅓ cup shredded **reduced-fat Mexican-blend cheese**
¼ cup chopped **scallions**

seasonings:
¼ teaspoon chili powder
¼ teaspoon ground cumin

293 CALORIES

You'll need: 8-inch by 8-inch baking pan, nonstick spray, medium bowl, large skillet, paper towels, foil

Prep: 10 minutes
Cook: 25 minutes

1. Preheat oven to 375 degrees. Spray an 8-inch by 8-inch baking pan with nonstick spray.

2. In a medium bowl, combine cream cheese with ¼ cup enchilada sauce. Mix until uniform.

3. Bring a large skillet sprayed with nonstick spray to medium heat. Add shrimp, and sprinkle with seasonings. Cook for about 2 minutes per side, until blackened and cooked through.

4. Roughly chop shrimp, and add to the medium bowl. Stir to coat.

5. Place tortillas between 2 damp paper towels. Microwave for 20 seconds, or until warm and pliable.

6. Top half of each tortilla with the saucy shrimp. Roll each tortilla up over the filling, and place in the baking pan, seam side down.

7. Top with remaining ¼ cup enchilada sauce. Cover pan with foil. Bake for 15 minutes.

8. Remove foil, and sprinkle with shredded cheese. Bake until melted, about 3 minutes.

9. Top with scallions.

MAKES 2 SERVINGS

SHRIMP & CAULI' GRITS

 Entire recipe: 307 calories, 15g total fat (8.5g sat fat), 637mg sodium, 19g carbs, 6g fiber, 7.5g sugars, 26.5g protein

6

2 cups **riced cauliflower**
2½ tablespoons **light/reduced-fat cream cheese**
2 teaspoons grated **Parmesan cheese**
2 teaspoons **whipped butter**
3 ounces (about 6) **raw large shrimp**, peeled, tails removed, deveined
1 teaspoon **lemon juice**

seasonings:
¼ teaspoon garlic powder
¼ teaspoon onion powder
⅛ teaspoon black pepper

307 CALORIES

You'll need: skillet with a lid, nonstick spray, medium bowl

Prep: 5 minutes
Cook: 10 minutes

1. Bring a skillet sprayed with nonstick spray to medium-high heat. Add cauliflower and 2 tablespoons water. Cover and cook for 3 minutes.

2. Uncover skillet. Cook and stir until cauliflower is tender and water has evaporated, about 1 minute.

3. Reduce heat to medium low. Add cream cheese, Parm, butter, and ⅛ teaspoon of each seasoning. Cook and stir until cream cheese and butter have melted and mixed, about 1 minute. Transfer to a medium bowl, and cover to keep warm.

4. Remove skillet from heat; clean, if needed. Respray, and bring to medium heat. Add shrimp, lemon juice, and remaining ⅛ teaspoon each garlic powder and onion powder. Cook and stir for about 4 minutes, until cooked through.

5. Serve shrimp over cauliflower grits.

MAKES 1 SERVING

EXTRA, EXTRA!

Top with chopped chives for extra yum!

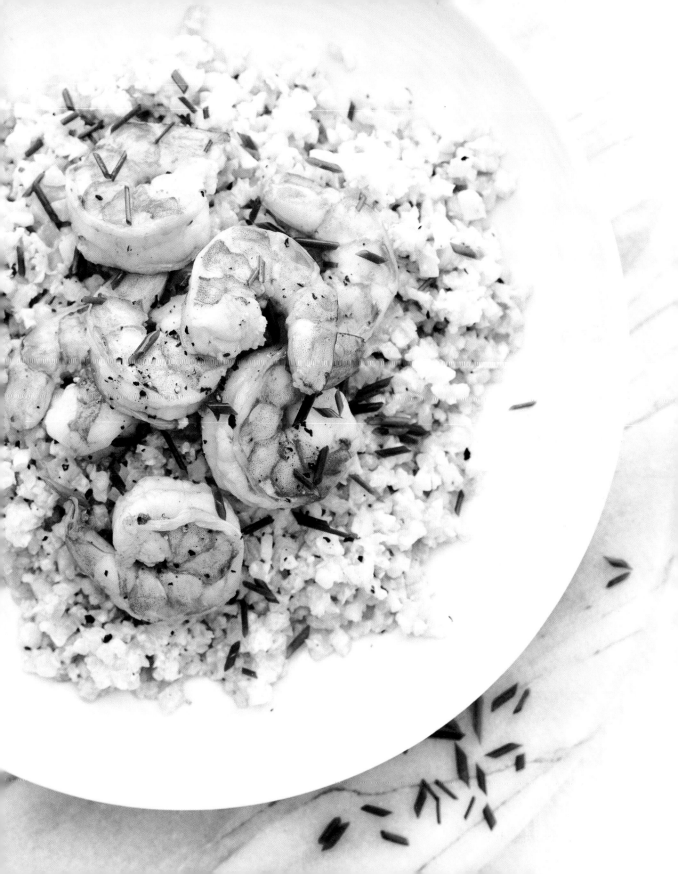

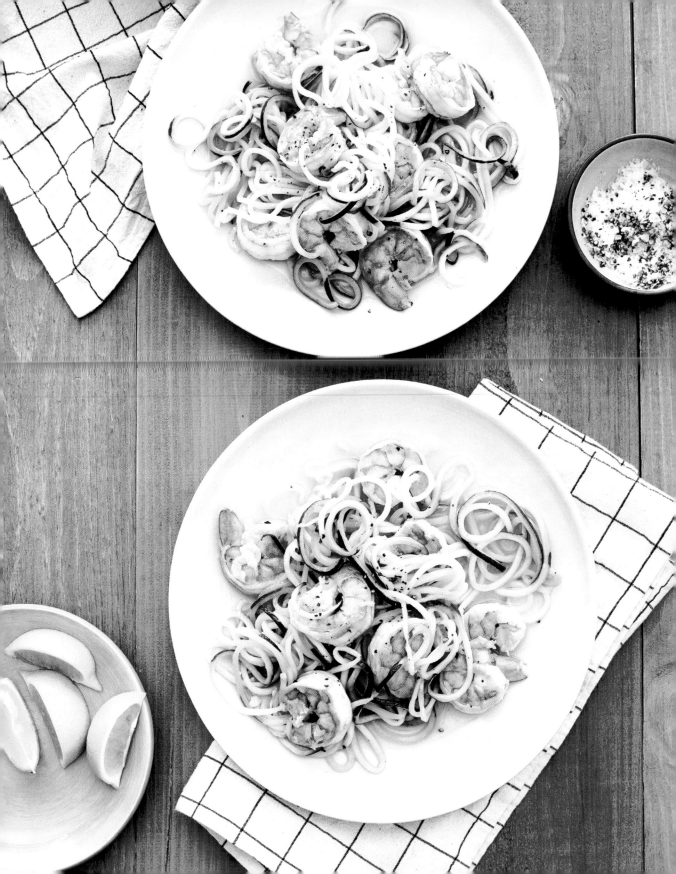

SHRIMP SCAMPI Z'PAGHETTI

½ of recipe (about 1½ cups): 274 calories, 9g total fat (4.5g sat fat), 709mg sodium, 21g carbs, 5g fiber, 12.5g sugars, 26g protein

1½ pounds (about 3 medium) **spiralized zucchini**
1 cup chopped **onion**
8 ounces (about 16) **raw large shrimp**, peeled, tails removed, deveined
2 tablespoons **dry white wine**
2 tablespoons **lemon juice**
2 tablespoons **whipped butter**

seasonings:
¾ teaspoon garlic powder
¼ teaspoon salt
⅛ teaspoon black pepper

You'll need: skillet, nonstick spray, strainer

Prep: 10 minutes
Cook: 15 minutes

HG FYI

Check out the Zucchini Noodles Made Simple guide on page 362.

1. Bring a skillet sprayed with nonstick spray to medium-high heat. Cook and stir zucchini until hot and slightly softened, about 3 minutes.

2. Transfer to a strainer, and thoroughly drain.

3. Remove skillet from heat, respray, and return to medium-high heat. Cook and stir onion until mostly softened and browned, about 5 minutes.

4. Add shrimp, wine, lemon juice, seasonings, and 1 tablespoon water. Cook and stir for about 4 minutes, until shrimp are cooked through and liquid has reduced.

5. Reduce heat to low. Add butter and drained zucchini. Cook and stir until zucchini is hot and butter has melted and mixed with sauce, about 2 minutes.

MAKES 2 SERVINGS

SALMON Z'PAGHETTI GIRLFREDO

30m **GF** **½ of recipe (1 fillet with about 1¼ cups noodles):** 301 calories, 16.5g total fat (6.5g sat fat), 536mg sodium, 9.5g carbs, 2.5g fiber, 6.5g sugars, 29g protein

6

1 pound (about 2 medium) **spiralized zucchini**
2½ tablespoons **light/reduced-fat cream cheese**
2 teaspoons **whipped butter**
2 teaspoons grated **Parmesan cheese**
1 teaspoon chopped **garlic**
Two 4-ounce **raw skinless salmon fillets**

seasonings:
½ teaspoon onion powder
¼ teaspoon each salt and black pepper

301 CALORIES

You'll need: large skillet, nonstick spray, strainer, large bowl

Prep: 10 minutes
Cook: 15 minutes

1. Bring a large skillet sprayed with nonstick spray to medium-high heat. Cook and stir zucchini until hot and slightly softened, about 3 minutes.

2. Transfer to a strainer, and thoroughly drain.

3. Remove skillet from heat, respray, and bring to medium-low heat. Add drained zucchini, cream cheese, butter, Parm, garlic, onion powder, and ⅛ teaspoon each salt and pepper. Cook and stir until sauce is uniform and has coated zucchini, about 2 minutes. Transfer to a large bowl, and cover to keep warm.

4. Remove skillet from heat; clean, if needed. Respray, and bring to medium heat. Season salmon with remaining ⅛ teaspoon each salt and pepper. Cook for about 3 minutes per side, until cooked through.

5. Serve salmon over zucchini.

MAKES 2 SERVINGS

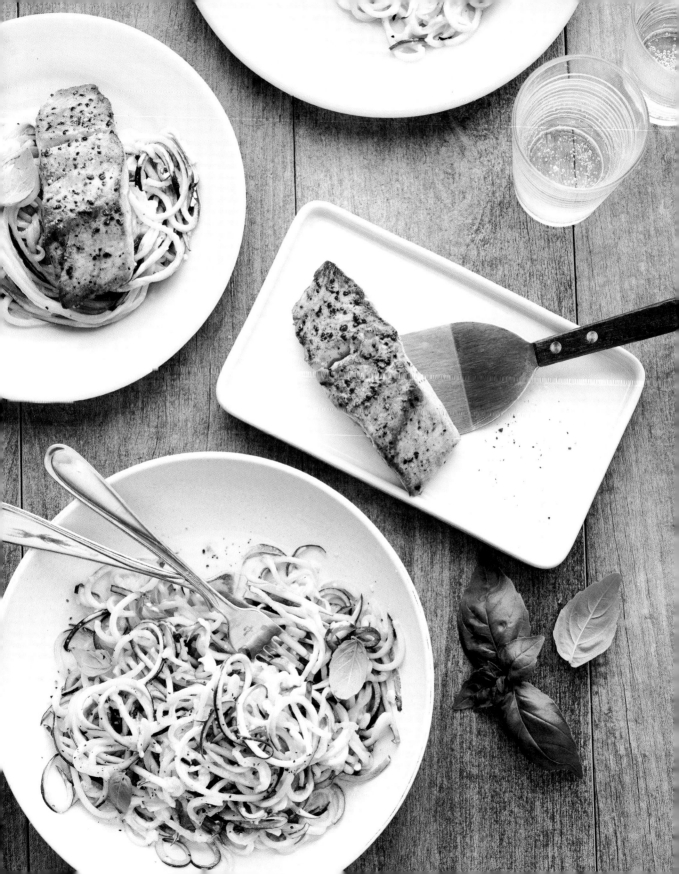

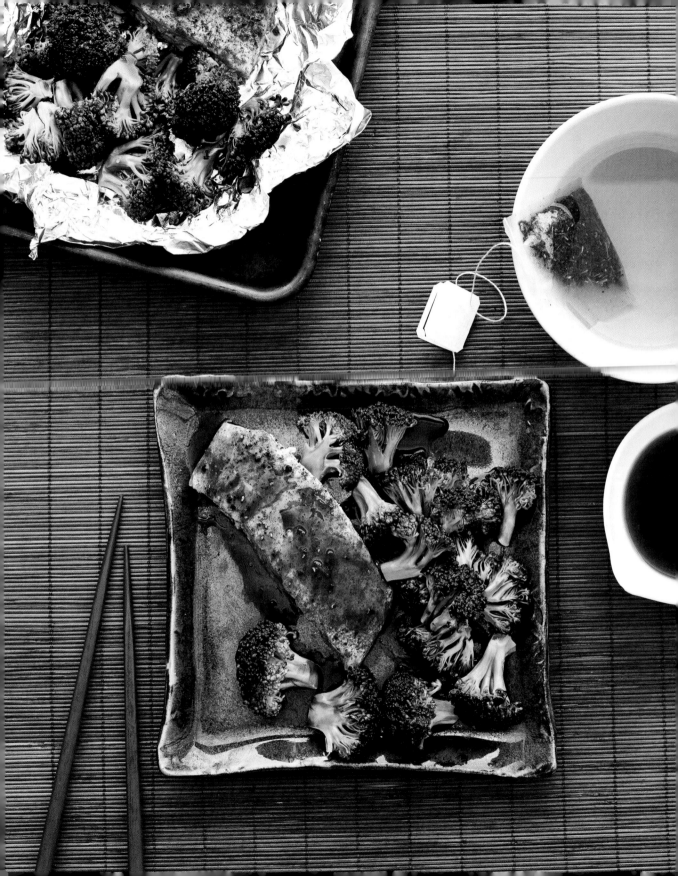

THAI OH MY SALMON & BROCCOLI

 30m **½ of recipe (1 fillet with about 1 cup broccoli):** 288 calories, 9.5g total fat (2.5g sat fat), 756mg sodium, 23g carbs, 3g fiber, 14.5g sugars, 27.5g protein

4

3 tablespoons **sweet Asian chili sauce**
1 tablespoon **reduced-sodium/lite soy sauce**
2½ cups **small broccoli florets**
Two 4-ounce **raw skinless salmon fillets**

seasonings:
¼ teaspoon garlic powder
⅛ teaspoon paprika

288 CALORIES

You'll need: heavy-duty foil, baking sheet, nonstick spray, small bowl

Prep: 10 minutes
Cook: 20 minutes

1. Preheat oven to 375 degrees. Lay a large piece of heavy-duty foil on a baking sheet, and spray with nonstick spray.

2. In a small bowl, combine chili sauce, soy sauce, and 2 teaspoons water. Mix until uniform.

3. Place broccoli on the center of the foil. Top with salmon, and sprinkle with seasonings. Drizzle with sauce mixture.

4. Cover with another large piece of foil. Fold together and seal all four edges of the foil pieces, forming a well-sealed packet.

5. Bake for 20 minutes, or until salmon is cooked through and broccoli is tender.

6. Cut packet to release hot steam before opening entirely.

MAKES 2 SERVINGS

SCOTT'S NUTTY AVOCADO SALMON

 ½ of recipe: 236 calories, 13.5g total fat (3g sat fat), 452mg sodium, 3g carbs, 2g fiber, 0.5g sugars, 25g protein

5

Two 4-ounce **raw skinless salmon fillets**
1¼ ounces (2 heaping tablespoons) mashed **avocado**
1½ teaspoons **fat-free milk**
⅛ teaspoon **lemon juice**
¼ ounce (about 1 tablespoon) sliced **almonds**

seasonings:
¼ teaspoon garlic powder
¼ teaspoon onion powder
¼ teaspoon plus a dash each salt and black pepper

236 CALORIES

You'll need: baking sheet, nonstick spray, small bowl

Prep: 5 minutes
Cook: 15 minutes

1. Preheat oven to 450 degrees. Spray a baking sheet with nonstick spray.

2. Season salmon with ⅛ teaspoon of each seasoning. Place on the baking sheet, and bake until cooked through, about 14 minutes.

3. In a small bowl, combine avocado, milk, lemon juice, remaining ⅛ teaspoon each garlic powder and onion powder, and remaining dash each salt and pepper. Mix until mostly smooth and uniform.

4. Spread over salmon, and sprinkle with almonds.

MAKES 2 SERVINGS

HG FYI

This recipe was inspired by Scott Wolf (the Hungry Girl fan, not the actor!). His favorite HG recipe is Shrimp & Grits . . . for Hungry Chicks! (Visit hungry-girl.com/grits for the recipe.)

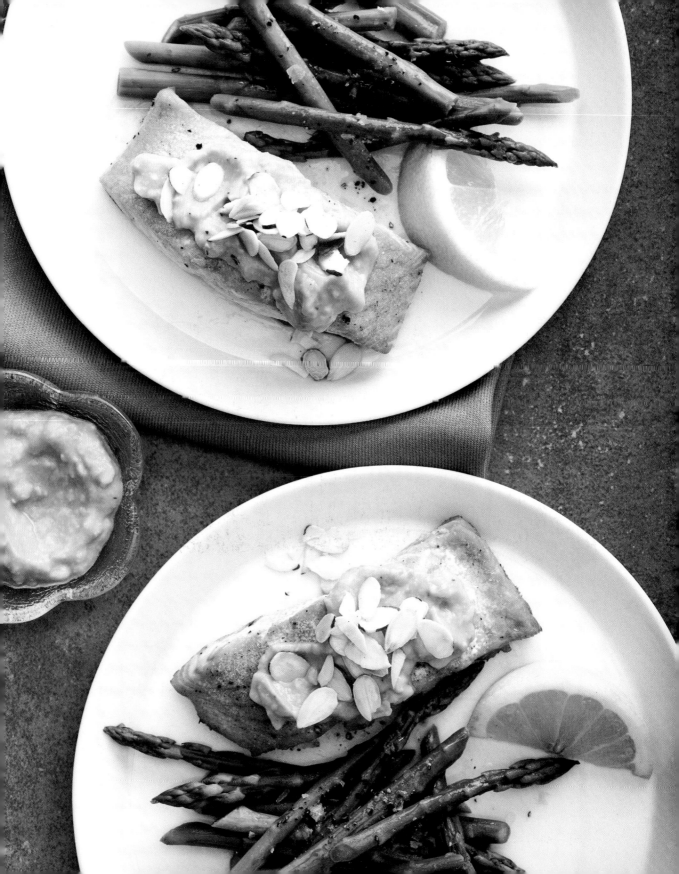

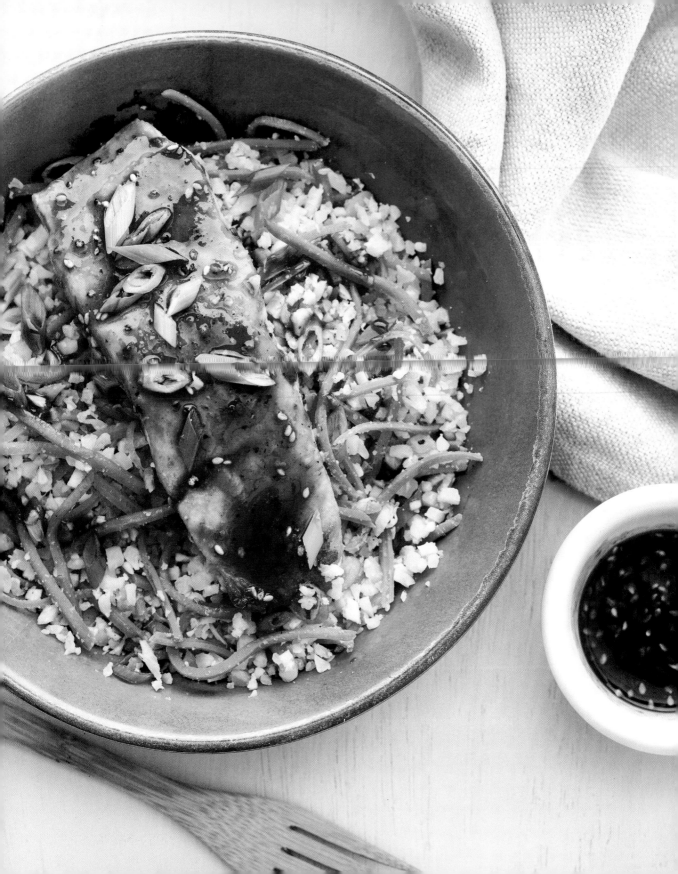

TERIYAKI SALMON CAULIFLOWER RICE BOWL

 Entire recipe: 298 calories, 10g total fat (2.5g sat fat), 590mg sodium, 25g carbs, 6.5g fiber, 11.5g sugars, 29g protein

5

1½ cups **riced cauliflower**
½ cup shredded **carrots**
3 tablespoons chopped **scallions**
4 ounces **raw skinless salmon fillet**
1 tablespoon **thick teriyaki sauce or marinade**

seasonings:
½ teaspoon plus ⅛ teaspoon garlic powder
½ teaspoon plus ⅛ teaspoon onion powder

You'll need: large skillet, nonstick spray, medium bowl, small bowl

Prep: 5 minutes
Cook: 15 minutes

1. Bring a large skillet sprayed with nonstick spray to medium-high heat. Add cauliflower, carrots, and ½ teaspoon of each seasoning. Cook and stir until softened, about 6 minutes.

2. Remove skillet from heat, and stir in 2 tablespoons scallions. Transfer to a medium bowl, and cover to keep warm.

3. Clean skillet, if needed. Respray, and return to medium-high heat. Season salmon with remaining ⅛ teaspoon of each seasoning. Cook for about 3 minutes per side, until cooked through.

4. In a small bowl, mix teriyaki with 1 teaspoon warm water.

5. Add salmon to the bowl of veggies, and drizzle with teriyaki mixture.

6. Top with remaining 1 tablespoon scallions.

MAKES 1 SERVING

TROPICAL FISH TACOS

 ½ of recipe (2 tacos): 243 calories, 3.5g total fat (0.5g sat fat), 284mg sodium, 28.5g carbs, 3.5g fiber, 7.5g sugars, 25g protein

6

¾ cup **shredded cabbage** or **bagged cole slaw mix**
¼ cup chopped **fresh cilantro**
1½ teaspoons **lime juice**
8 ounces raw **tilapia**
Four **6-inch corn tortillas**
½ cup **chopped mango**

seasonings:
Dash plus ⅛ teaspoon salt
Dash black pepper
½ teaspoon taco seasoning

243 CALORIES

You'll need: small bowl, skillet, nonstick spray, paper towels

Prep: 10 minutes
Cook: 10 minutes

1. In a small bowl, combine cabbage/slaw mix, cilantro, lime juice, and a dash each salt and pepper. Mix well.

2. Bring a skillet sprayed with nonstick spray to medium-high heat. Season tilapia with taco seasoning and remaining ⅛ teaspoon salt. Cook for 2 minutes per side, or until cooked through.

3. Wrap tortillas in 2 damp paper towels, and microwave for 20 seconds, or until warm.

4. Evenly distribute slaw mixture among tortillas, followed by tilapia.

5. Top with mango.

MAKES 2 SERVINGS

HG TIPS

- **Whip up some extra slaw to serve on the side!**

- **For a flavor boost, char tortillas in a dry skillet over high heat!**

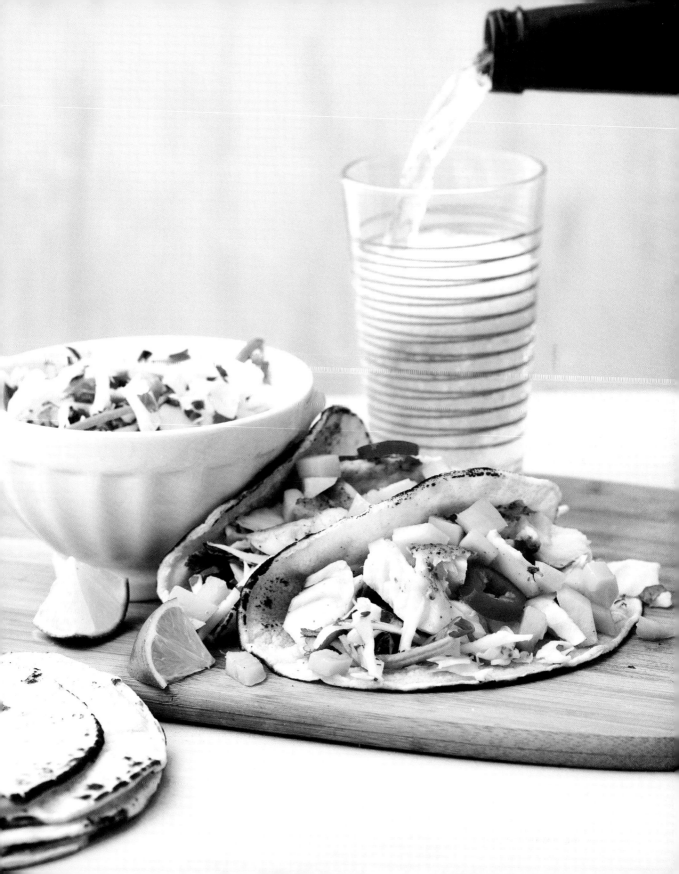

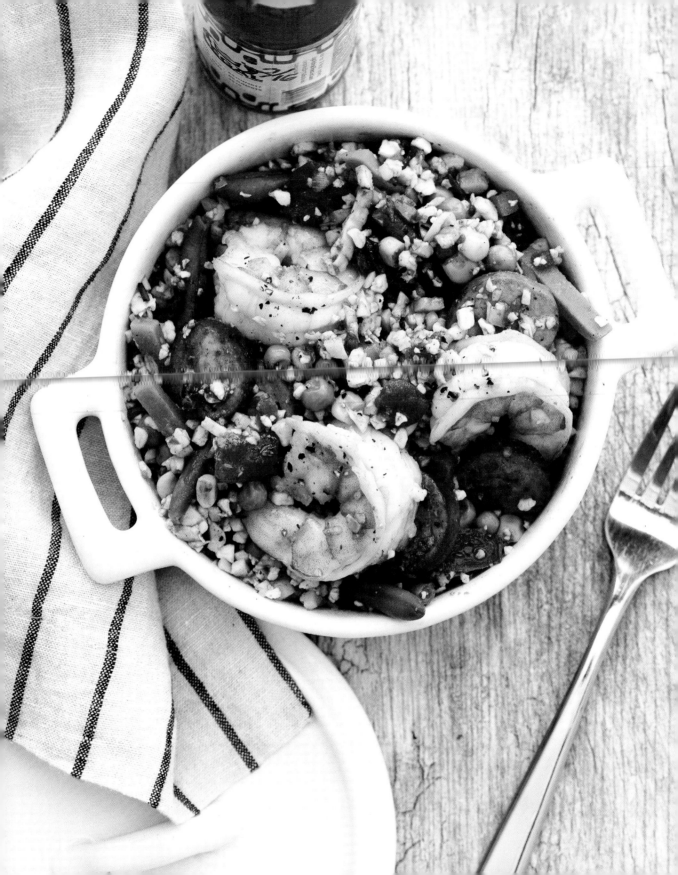

SKILLET JAMBALAYA

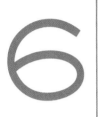 **GF** **⅙th of recipe (about 1⅓ cups):** 152 calories, 3g total fat (1g sat fat), 656mg sodium, 17g carbs, 4.5g fiber, 6.5g sugars, 14g protein

6

5 cups **riced cauliflower**
3 cups **frozen petite mixed vegetables**
One 14.5-ounce can **fire-roasted diced tomatoes** (not drained)
6 ounces (about 2 links) **fully cooked chicken sausage**, sliced into coins
1 tablespoon chopped **garlic**
6 ounces (about 12) **raw large shrimp**, peeled, tails removed, deveined

seasonings:
2 teaspoons Cajun seasoning
½ teaspoon dried oregano
¼ teaspoon salt
⅛ teaspoon cayenne pepper

152
CALORIES

You'll need: extra-large skillet, nonstick spray

Prep: 10 minutes
Cook: 20 minutes

1. Bring an extra-large skillet sprayed with nonstick spray to medium-high heat. Add all ingredients and seasonings *except* shrimp. Cook and stir until cauliflower has softened and frozen veggies have thawed, 10 to 12 minutes.

2. Add shrimp. Cook and stir for about 4 minutes, until shrimp are cooked through and entire dish is hot.

MAKES 6 SERVINGS

HG FYI

Get the 411 on riced cauliflower . . .
See page 365.

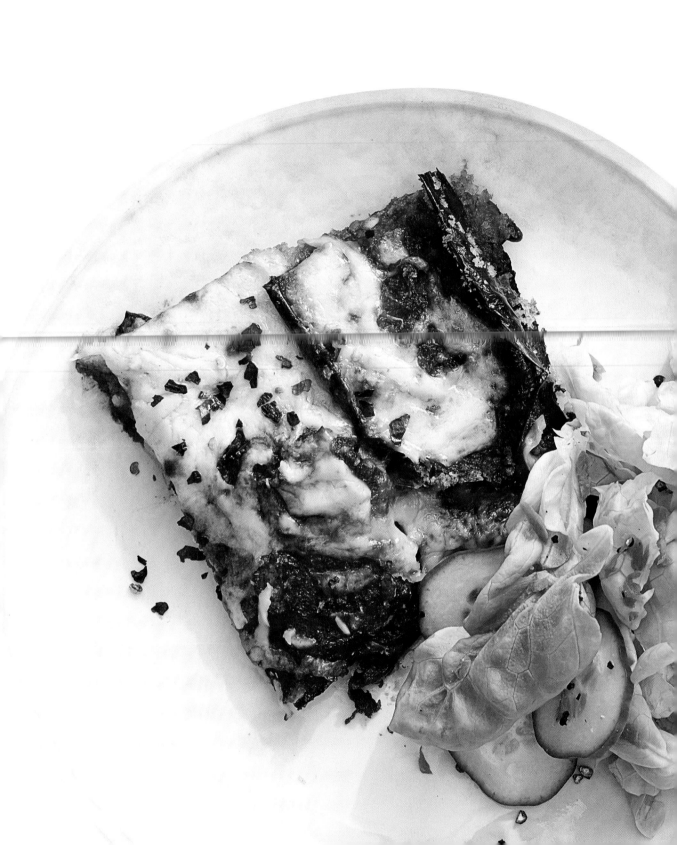

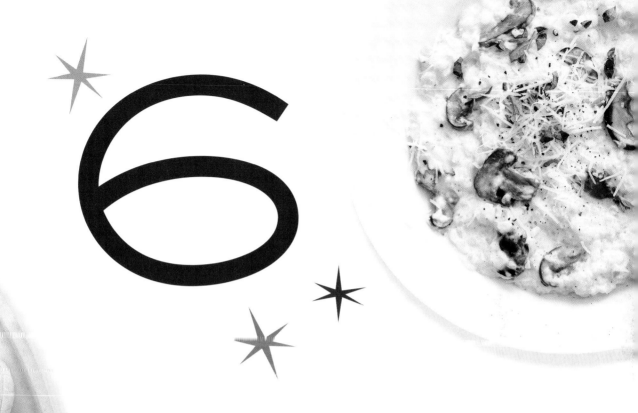

6

SIMPLY VEGGIE

From meals that just don't contain meat, to recipes PACKED with veggies, this chapter has it all! Pasta swaps, pizza, cauliflower rice, and more . . .

SPICY SLOW-COOKER VEGGIE CHILI

(V) (GF) **⅕th of recipe (about 1 cup):** 163 calories, 0.5g total fat (0g sat fat), 722mg sodium, 32g carbs, 9g fiber, 10g sugars, 8.5g protein

One 29-ounce can **crushed tomatoes**
One 15-ounce can **red kidney beans**, drained and rinsed
1½ cups chopped **brown mushrooms**
1 cup chopped **onion**
1 cup chopped **bell pepper**
⅓ cup **jarred jalapeño slices**, drained and chopped

seasonings:
1 tablespoon chili seasoning mix

163 CALORIES

You'll need: slow cooker

Prep: 10 minutes
Cook: 3 to 4 hours or 7 to 8 hours

1. Add ingredients and seasoning to a slow cooker, and thoroughly stir.

2. Cover and cook on high for 3 to 4 hours or on low for 7 to 8 hours.

MAKES 5 SERVINGS

HG FYI

Chili seasoning is one of my go-to pantry staples. For a DIY version, flip to page 357.

SURVEY SAYS . . .

56% of Hungry Girl fans like their chili spicy. The rest of you can leave out the jalapeños in this recipe!

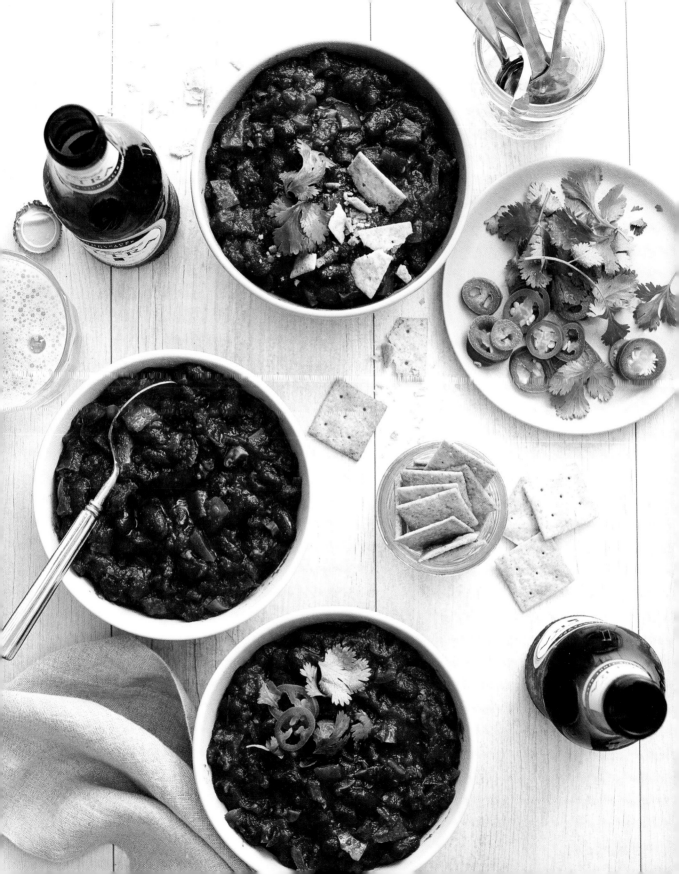

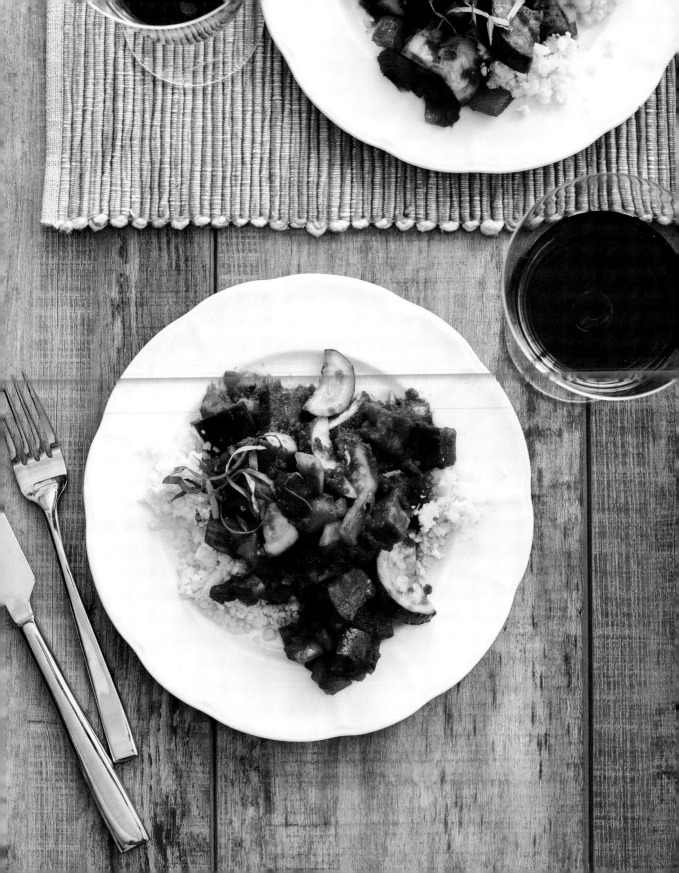

SHEET-PAN RATATOUILLE

 **½ of recipe (about 2 cups):** 162 calories, 0.5g fat (<0.5g sat fat), 356mg sodium, 34.5g carbs, 9.5g fiber, 19g sugars, 7g protein

6

1½ cups cubed **eggplant**
1 cup chopped **red bell pepper**
1 cup sliced and halved **zucchini**
1 cup **canned fire-roasted diced tomatoes**, drained
⅔ cup roughly chopped **onion**
½ cup **tomato paste**

seasonings:
2 teaspoons dried basil
½ teaspoon garlic powder
½ teaspoon onion powder

162 CALORIES

You'll need:
baking sheet, nonstick spray, large bowl, foil

Prep: 10 minutes
Cook: 30 minutes

1. Preheat oven to 375 degrees. Spray a baking sheet with nonstick spray.

2. Place ingredients and seasonings in a large bowl, and stir until uniform.

3. Distribute mixture onto the center of the baking sheet. Cover with a large piece of foil.

4. Bake for 30 minutes, or until veggies are tender.

5. Carefully release steam before uncovering entirely.

MAKES 2 SERVINGS

EXTRA, EXTRA!

I love this served over riced cauliflower . . .
Mmmm! Flip to page 365 for DIY tips!

SHEET-PAN ROASTED VEGGIES

V **GF** **¼th of recipe (about 1 cup):** 128 calories, 3.5g total fat (0.5g sat fat), 144mg sodium, 23.5g carbs, 6g fiber, 8.5g sugars, 2g protein

5

2 cups (about ½ of a medium) peeled **butternut squash** cut into 1-inch chunks

1 cup (about 2 medium) peeled **carrots** cut into 1-inch chunks

1 cup (about 1 medium) peeled **parsnip** cut into 1-inch chunks

1 cup (1 to 2 medium) peeled **beets** cut into 1-inch chunks

1 tablespoon **olive oil**

seasonings:
⅛ teaspoon each salt and black pepper

128 CALORIES

You'll need: baking sheet, nonstick spray, large bowl

Prep: 20 minutes
Cook: 35 minutes

1. Preheat oven to 400 degrees. Spray a baking sheet with nonstick spray.

2. Place veggies in a large bowl. Drizzle with oil, and sprinkle with salt and pepper. Gently toss to coat.

3. Evenly distribute mixture on the baking sheet. Bake for 15 minutes.

4. Flip veggies. Bake until softened and browned, 18 to 20 minutes.

MAKES 4 SERVINGS

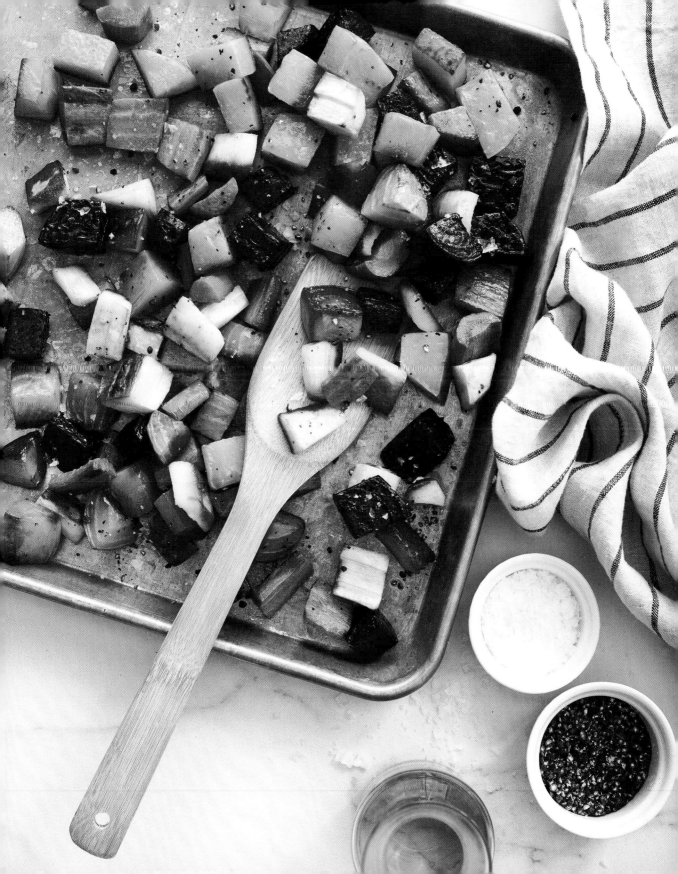

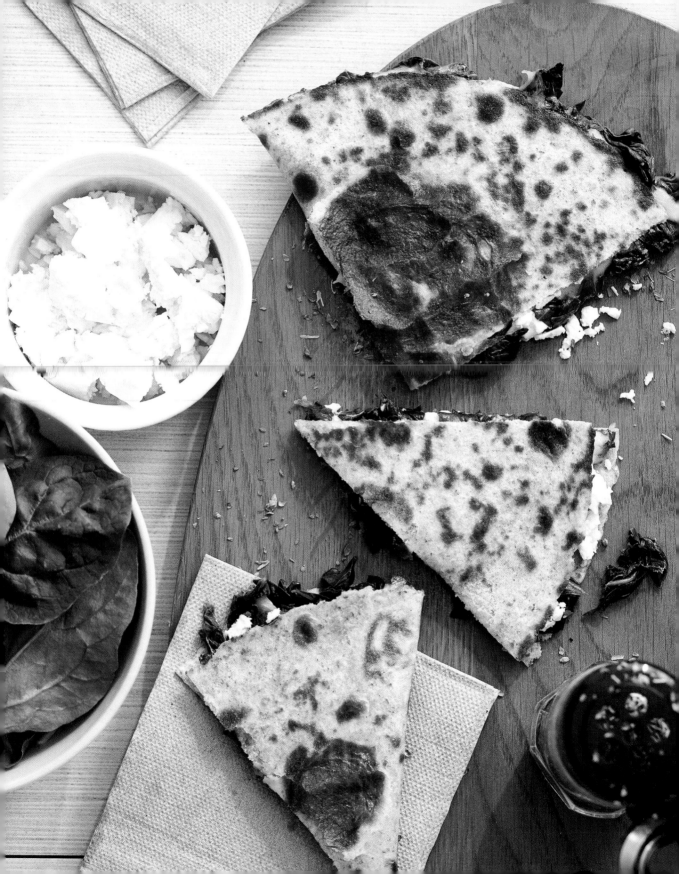

SPINACH-FETA QUESADILLA

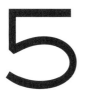 **Entire recipe:** 253 calories, 10.5g total fat (6g sat fat), 742mg sodium, 29.5g carbs, 8g fiber, 1.5g sugars, 18g protein

5

3 cups chopped **spinach**
1 teaspoon chopped **garlic**
2 tablespoons crumbled **feta cheese**
1 **large high-fiber flour tortilla** with 110 calories or less
¼ cup shredded **part-skim mozzarella cheese**

seasonings:
¼ teaspoon Italian seasoning

You'll need: large skillet, nonstick spray, medium bowl

Prep: 5 minutes
Cook: 10 minutes

1. Bring a large skillet sprayed with nonstick spray to medium-high heat. Add spinach, garlic, and Italian seasoning. Cook and stir until wilted, about 2 minutes. Stir in feta, and transfer to a medium bowl.

2. Remove skillet from heat; clean, if needed. Respray and bring to medium heat. Add tortilla, and top with mozzarella. Spoon spinach mixture over half of the tortilla. Cook until mozzarella has melted, about 2 minutes.

3. Using a spatula, fold the cheese-only tortilla half over the filling, and press lightly to seal. Carefully flip and cook until crispy, about 2 minutes.

4. Slice into wedges.

MAKES 1 SERVING

SPICY SOFRITAS TACOS

 V **GF** **½ of recipe (2 tacos):** 294 calories, 11g total fat (2.5g sat fat), 463mg sodium, 28.5g carbs, 4.5g fiber, 3.5g sugars, 19.5g protein

6

½ cup chopped **tomatoes**
2 tablespoons **canned chipotle peppers in adobo sauce**
8 ounces **block-style extra-firm tofu**
Four **6-inch corn tortillas**
½ cup shredded **lettuce**
¼ cup shredded **reduced-fat Mexican blend cheese**

seasonings:
2 teaspoons taco seasoning

294 CALORIES

You'll need: small blender or food processor, skillet, nonstick spray, paper towels

Prep: 10 minutes
Cook: 10 minutes

1. To make the sauce, place ¼ cup tomatoes in a small blender or food processor. Add peppers in adobo sauce, 1 teaspoon taco seasoning, and ¼ cup water. Blend until smooth.

2. Bring a skillet sprayed with nonstick spray to medium heat. Add tofu and remaining 1 teaspoon taco seasoning. Cook and crumble until lightly browned, about 3 minutes.

3. Add sauce, and cook and stir until hot and well mixed, about 1 minute.

4. Wrap tortillas in damp paper towels, and microwave for 20 seconds, or until warm.

5. Evenly distribute tofu mixture among tortillas. Top with lettuce, cheese, and remaining ¼ cup tomatoes.

MAKES 2 SERVINGS

EXTRA, EXTRA!

A squeeze of lime juice adds bonus flavor. Jalapeños bring some heat!

HG TIP

For a flavor boost, char your tortillas in a dry skillet over high heat.

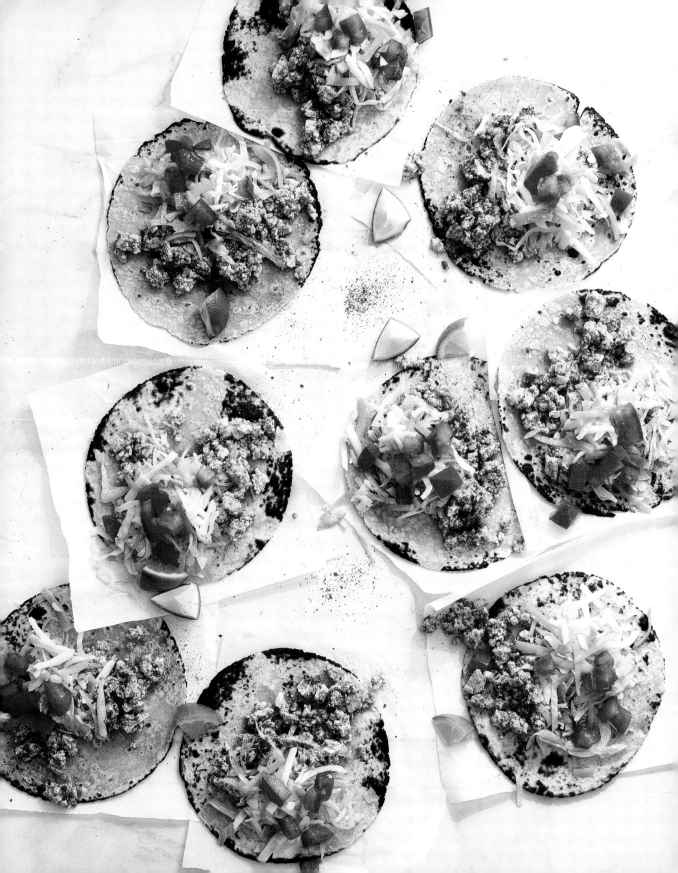

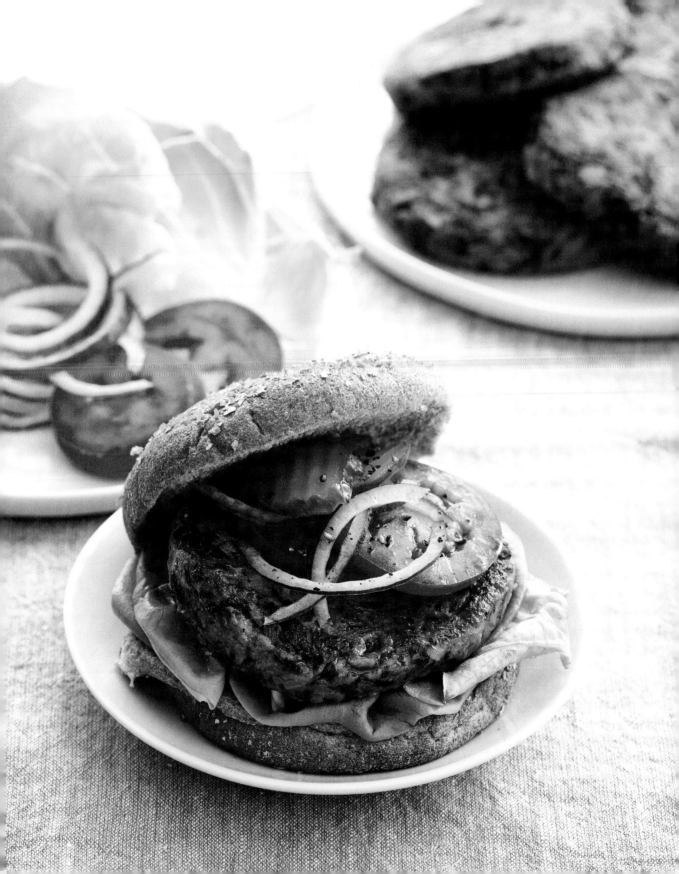

BUTTERNUT VEGGIE BURGERS

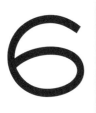

V **⅙th of recipe (1 patty):** 144 calories, 1g total fat (0g sat fat), 493mg sodium, 27g carbs, 6.5g fiber, 3.5g sugars, 7.5g protein

3 cups cubed **butternut squash**
1 cup finely chopped **onion**
One 15-ounce can **garbanzo beans** (a.k.a. chickpeas), drained and rinsed
¼ cup (about 2 large) **egg whites** or **fat-free liquid egg substitute**
One 10-ounce package **frozen spinach**, thawed, drained, and thoroughly patted dry
¼ cup **whole-wheat flour**

seasonings:
¾ teaspoon salt
½ teaspoon garlic powder
¼ teaspoon black pepper

144 CALORIES

You'll need: large skillet with lid, nonstick spray, large bowl, paper towels, small blender or food processor, potato masher

Prep: 15 minutes
Cook: 35 minutes

1. Bring a large skillet sprayed with nonstick spray to medium-high heat. Add squash, onion, ¼ teaspoon salt, ¼ teaspoon garlic powder, and ¼ cup water. Cover and cook for 8 minutes, or until squash has mostly softened and water has evaporated. Transfer to a large bowl lined with paper towels.

2. Place rinsed beans and egg in a small blender or food processor, and puree until mostly smooth.

3. Remove paper towels from veggie bowl, and blot away excess moisture. Roughly mash squash. Add bean puree, spinach, flour, remaining ½ teaspoon salt, remaining ¼ teaspoon garlic powder, and black pepper. Mix thoroughly.

4. Once cool, evenly form mixture into 6 patties, about ½ cup each.

5. If needed, clean skillet. Respray and bring to medium heat.

6. Working in batches, cook patties until firm and lightly browned, 3 to 4 minutes per side, flipping gently.

MAKES 6 SERVINGS

HG TIP

Flip to page 173 for my burger must-haves!

EASY EGGPLANT PARM

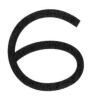 **¼th of recipe:** 254 calories, 9.5g total fat (5g sat fat), 685mg sodium, 25.5g carbs, 6.5g fiber, 9.5g sugars, 18.5g protein

6

¾ cup **whole-wheat panko breadcrumbs**
½ cup (about 4 large) **egg whites** or **fat-free liquid egg substitute**
1 large **eggplant** (about 20 ounces), ends removed
1 cup **marinara sauce** with 3g fat or less per serving
1 cup shredded **part-skim mozzarella cheese**
¼ cup grated **Parmesan cheese**

seasonings:
½ teaspoon garlic powder
½ teaspoon onion powder
⅛ teaspoon each salt and black pepper

You'll need: baking sheet, 8-inch by 8-inch baking pan, nonstick spray, two wide bowls, foil

Prep: 20 minutes
Cook: 1 hour 5 minutes
Cool: 10 minutes

1. Preheat oven to 400 degrees. Spray a baking sheet and an 8-inch by 8-inch baking pan with nonstick spray.

2. In a wide bowl, mix breadcrumbs with seasonings. Place egg in a second wide bowl.

3. Cut eggplant lengthwise into ½-inch slices.

4. One at a time, lightly coat eggplant slices with egg, shake to remove excess, coat with seasoned crumbs, and place on the baking sheet.

5. Top with any excess breadcrumbs. Bake for 20 minutes.

6. Flip eggplant. Bake until slightly softened and lightly browned, about 10 minutes.

7. In the baking pan, evenly layer ¼ cup marinara, half of the eggplant, ¼ cup marinara, ½ cup mozzarella, 2 tablespoons Parm, and ¼ cup marinara. Continue layering with remaining eggplant slices, ¼ cup marinara, ½ cup mozzarella, and 2 tablespoons Parm.

8. Cover with foil. Bake for 30 minutes, or until hot and bubbly.

9. Uncover and bake until cheese has melted and lightly browned, about 5 minutes.

10. Let cool for 10 minutes before slicing.

MAKES 4 SERVINGS

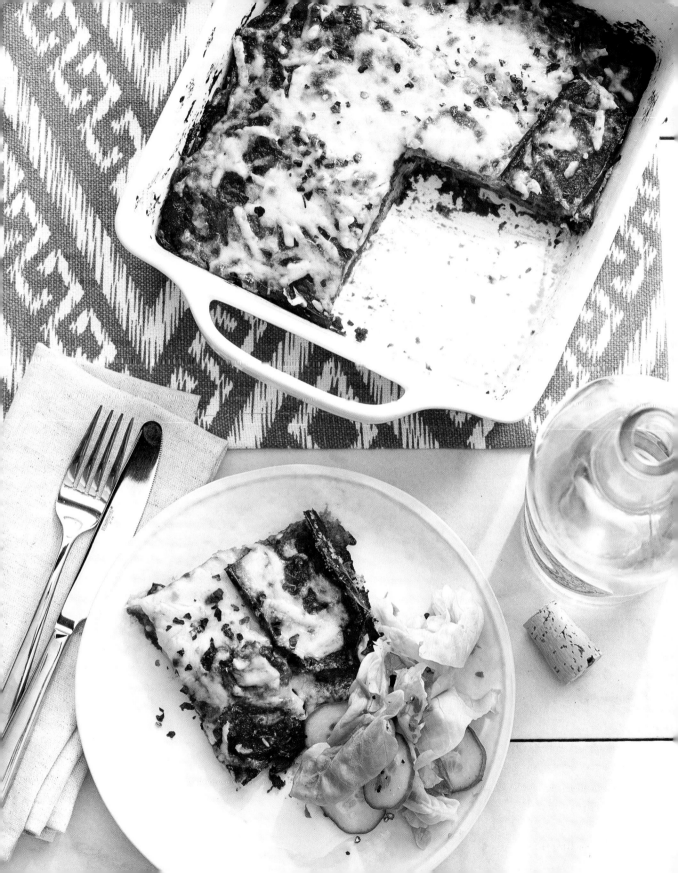

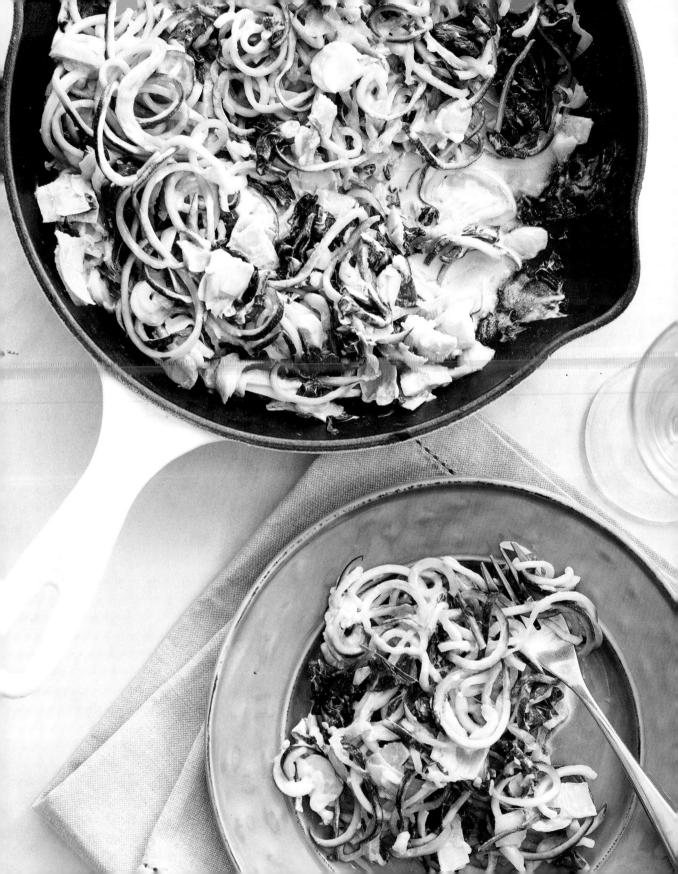

SPINACH & ARTICHOKE Z'PAGHETTI

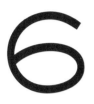

¼th of recipe (about 1¼ cups): 166 calories, 7.5g total fat (4g sat fat), 489mg sodium, 15.5g carbs, 5g fiber, 10g sugars, 12g protein

2 pounds (about 4 medium) **spiralized zucchini**
6 cups chopped **spinach**
1 cup **artichoke hearts packed in water**, thoroughly drained and chopped
½ cup **light sour cream**
½ cup shredded **part-skim mozzarella cheese**
2 tablespoons grated **Parmesan cheese**

seasonings:
1 teaspoon garlic powder
Dash each salt and black pepper

166 CALORIES

You'll need: extra-large skillet, nonstick spray, strainer

Prep: 10 minutes
Cook: 10 minutes

1. Bring an extra-large skillet sprayed with nonstick spray to medium-high heat. Cook and stir zucchini until slightly softened, about 4 minutes.

2. Transfer zucchini to a strainer, and thoroughly drain excess liquid.

3. Respray skillet, and return to medium-high heat.

4. Add spinach, chopped artichoke hearts, and seasonings. Cook and stir until spinach has wilted and artichoke hearts are hot, about 2 minutes. Add drained zucchini.

5. Reduce heat to medium low. Add sour cream, mozzarella, and Parm. Cook and stir until hot and well mixed, about 2 minutes.

MAKES 4 SERVINGS

SESAME PEANUT ZOODLES

 ½ of recipe (about 1½ cups): 230 calories, 9g total fat (1g sat fat), 702mg sodium, 32.5g carbs, 6g fiber, 23.5g sugars, 9g protein

5

1½ pounds (about 3 medium) **spiralized zucchini**
1 cup shredded **carrot**
½ cup **Thai peanut sauce/salad dressing** with 60 calories or less per 2-tablespoon serving
¼ cup chopped **scallions**
2 teaspoons **sesame seeds**

You'll need: extra-large skillet, nonstick spray, strainer

Prep: 5 minutes
Cook: 10 minutes

1. Bring an extra-large skillet sprayed with nonstick spray to medium-high heat. Add zucchini and carrot. Cook and stir until hot and slightly softened, about 3 minutes.

2. Transfer to a strainer, and thoroughly drain.

3. Remove skillet from heat, respray, and return to medium-high heat. Return veggies, and cook and stir for 2 minutes.

4. Add sauce/dressing and scallions. Cook and stir until hot and well mixed, about 2 more minutes.

5. Serve topped with sesame seeds.

MAKES 2 SERVINGS

HG FYI

Spiralize your own zucchini, or grab premade noodles at the store . . . Details on page 362!

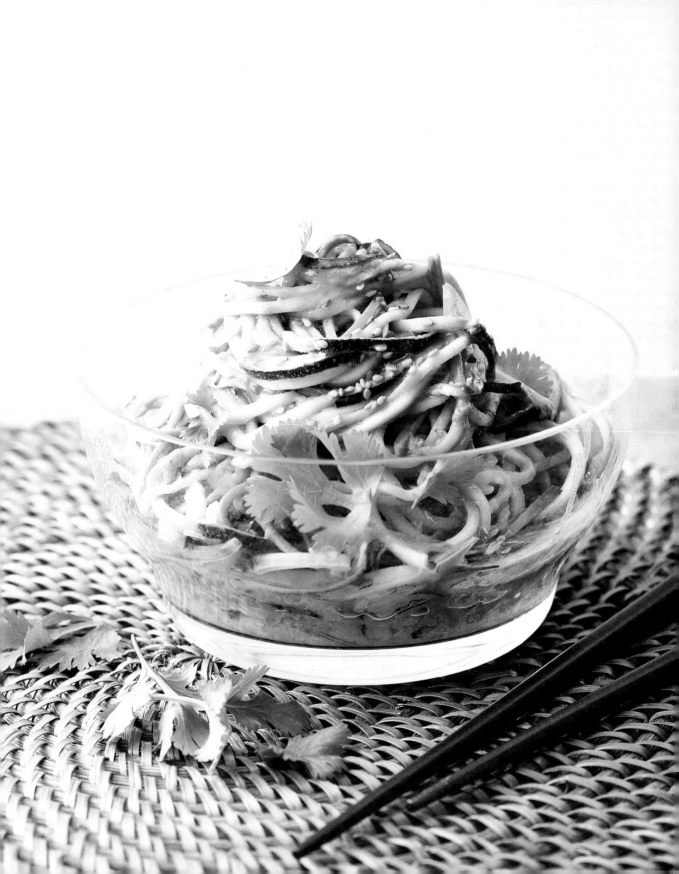

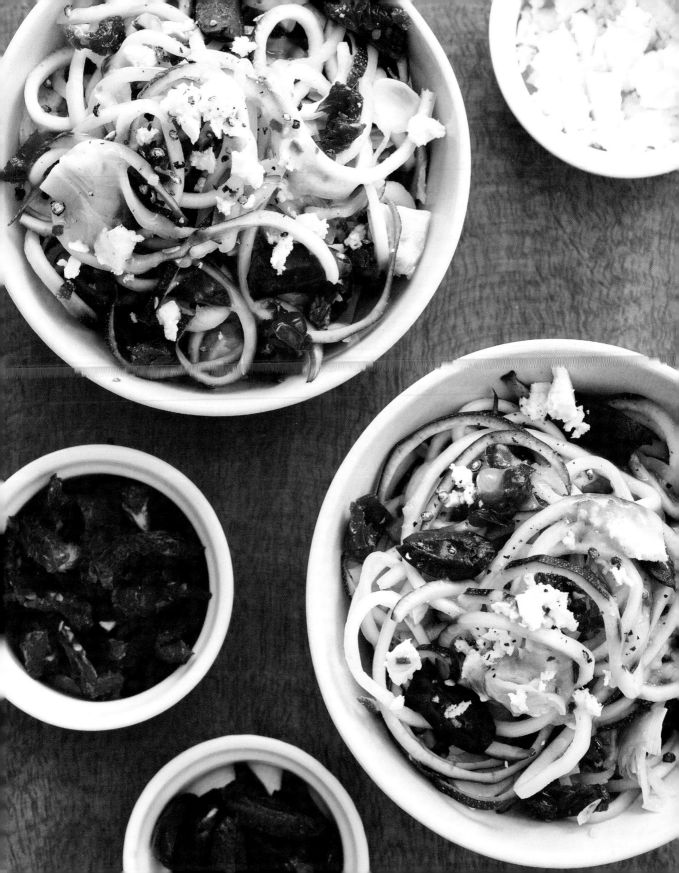

GREEK Z'PAGHETTI

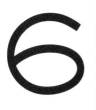 **½ of recipe (about 1½ cups):** 174 calories, 5.5g total fat (1.5g sat fat), 593mg sodium, 24.5g carbs, 7g fiber, 15g sugars, 8g protein

6

- 1½ pounds (about 3 medium) **spiralized zucchini**
- ½ cup **artichoke hearts packed in water**, drained and chopped
- ¼ cup bagged **sun-dried tomatoes** (not packed in oil), chopped
- 2 tablespoons sliced **Kalamata or black olives**
- 2 tablespoons **light Italian dressing**
- 2 tablespoons crumbled **feta cheese**

seasonings:
- ½ teaspoon garlic powder
- ½ teaspoon onion powder
- ¼ teaspoon dried oregano

You'll need: extra-large skillet, nonstick spray, strainer

Prep: 10 minutes
Cook: 5 minutes

1. Bring an extra-large skillet sprayed with nonstick spray to medium-high heat. Cook and stir zucchini until hot and slightly softened, about 3 minutes.

2. Transfer zucchini to a strainer, and thoroughly drain excess liquid.

3. Remove skillet from heat. Respray, and bring to medium heat. Add drained zucchini and all remaining ingredients and seasonings *except* feta. Cook and stir until entire dish is hot, about 2 minutes.

4. Serve topped with feta.

MAKES 2 SERVINGS

EZ ZOODLE LOW MEIN

 ½ of recipe (about 2½ cups): 139 calories, 1g total fat (<0.5g sat fat), 748mg sodium, 24g carbs, 6.5g fiber, 14.5g sugars, 8.5g protein

5

2 tablespoons **reduced-sodium/lite soy sauce**
1 teaspoon chopped **garlic**
3 cups **frozen Asian-style stir-fry vegetables**
1 cup quartered **mushrooms**
1½ pounds (about 3 medium) **spiralized zucchini**

seasonings:
¼ teaspoon ground ginger
¼ teaspoon onion powder
⅛ teaspoon salt

You'll need: small bowl, wok (or large skillet), nonstick spray, strainer

Prep: 10 minutes
Cook: 15 minutes

1. To make the sauce, in a small bowl, combine soy sauce, garlic, and seasonings. Mix well.

2. Bring a wok (or large skillet) sprayed with nonstick spray to medium-high heat. Add frozen veggies and mushrooms. Cook and stir until frozen veggies are hot and mushrooms have softened, about 5 minutes.

3. Add zucchini. Cook and stir until hot and slightly softened, about 3 minutes.

4. Transfer veggies to a strainer, and thoroughly drain excess liquid.

5. Return wok to medium-high heat, and add drained veggies. Add sauce, and cook and stir until evenly distributed and mostly absorbed, about 2 minutes.

MAKES 2 SERVINGS

HG FYI

I call this "low" mein because it's so low in calories!

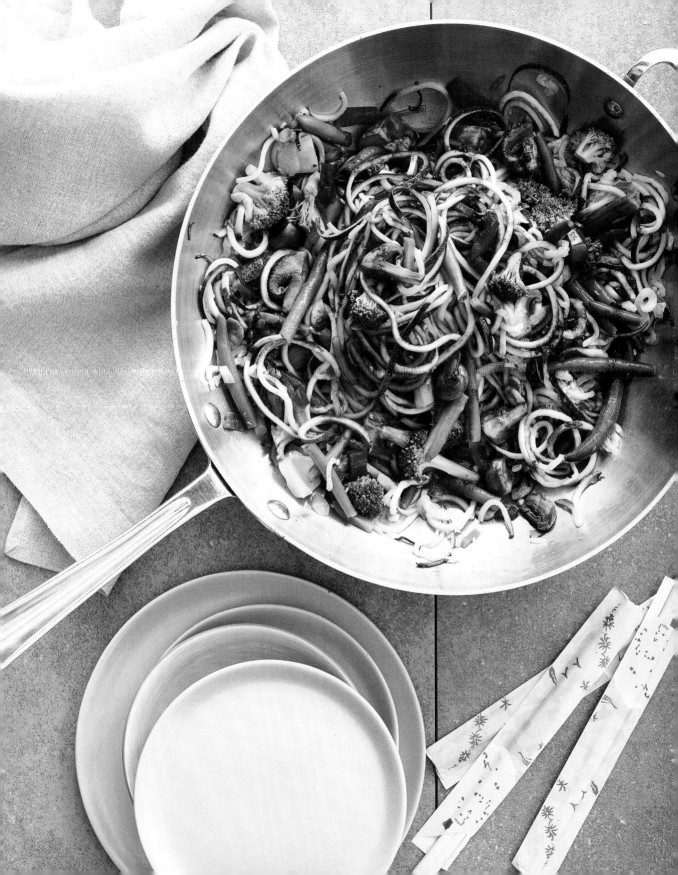

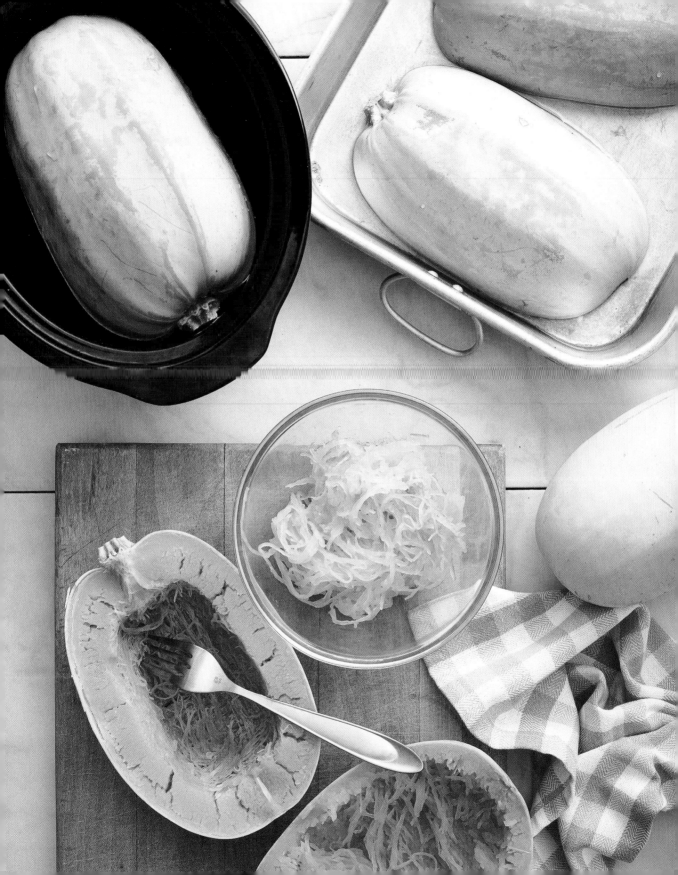

SLOW-COOKER SPAGHETTI SQUASH

V **GF** **1 cup cooked strands:** 42 calories, <0.5g total fat (0g sat fat), 28mg sodium, 10g carbs, 2g fiber, 4g sugars, 1g protein

1 | 1 **spaghetti squash** (about 4 pounds)

42 CALORIES

You'll need: slow cooker

Prep: 10 minutes
Cook: 2½ hours on high

1. Place whole squash in a slow cooker with ½ cup water. Cover and cook on high for 2½ hours or until squash is soft.

2. Once cool enough to handle, halve lengthwise; scoop out and discard seeds.

MAKES 5 OR MORE SERVINGS

INSTANT-POT SPAGHETTI SQUASH

V **GF** **1 cup cooked strands:** 42 calories, <0.5g total fat (0g sat fat), 28mg sodium, 10g carbs, 2g fiber, 4g sugars, 1g protein

1 | 1 **spaghetti squash** (about 4 pounds)

42 CALORIES

You'll need: Instant Pot

Prep: 15 minutes
Cook: 25 minutes

1. Microwave squash for 6 minutes, or until soft enough to cut.

2. Once cool enough to handle, halve lengthwise. Scoop out and discard seeds.

3. Place spaghetti squash halves on top of each other in the Instant Pot, cut sides up, and add 1 cup water.

4. Seal with lid. Set for 8 minutes.

5. Press Keep Warm/Cancel. Vent to release steam.

MAKES 5 OR MORE SERVINGS

OVEN-BAKED SPAGHETTI SQUASH

V **GF** **1 cup cooked strands:** 42 calories, <0.5g total fat (0g sat fat), 28mg sodium, 10g carbs, 2g fiber, 4g sugars, 1g protein

1 | 1 **spaghetti squash** (about 4 pounds)

42 CALORIES

You'll need: large baking pan

Prep: 15 minutes
Cook: 50 minutes

1. Preheat oven to 400 degrees.

2. Microwave squash for 6 minutes, or until soft enough to cut.

3. Once cool enough to handle, halve lengthwise. Scoop out and discard seeds.

4. Fill a large baking pan with ½ inch water, and place squash halves in the pan, cut sides down.

5. Bake until tender, about 40 minutes.

MAKES 5 OR MORE SERVINGS

HG FYI

A 4-pound squash yields about 5 cups cooked squash . . . sometimes more! The number of servings this recipe makes will vary based on your individual squash's size and yield.

SPEEDY SPAGHETTI SQUASH

 1 cup cooked strands: 42 calories, <0.5g total fat (0g sat fat), 28mg sodium, 10g carbs, 2g fiber, 4g sugars, 1g protein

1 | 1 **spaghetti squash** (about 4 pounds)

You'll need: extra-large microwave-safe bowl

Prep: 15 minutes
Cook: 20 minutes

1. Microwave squash for 6 minutes, or until soft enough to cut.

2. Once cool enough to handle, halve lengthwise. Scoop out and discard seeds.

3. Place one squash half in an extra-large microwave-safe bowl, cut side down. Add ¼ cup water. Cover and cook for 7 minutes, or until soft.

4. Repeat with remaining squash half.

MAKES 5 OR MORE SERVINGS

THREE-CHEESE SPAGHETTI SQUASH

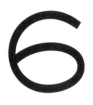 **½ of recipe (about 1⅓ cups):** 211 calories, 12.5g total fat (7.5g sat fat), 636mg sodium, 18.5g carbs, 3.5g fiber, 7g sugars, 9g protein

211 CALORIES

6

¼ cup shredded **reduced-fat cheddar cheese**

3 tablespoons **light/reduced-fat cream cheese**

1 tablespoon grated **Parmesan cheese**, or more for topping

1 tablespoon **whipped butter**

1½ teaspoons chopped **garlic**

3 cups **cooked spaghetti squash**, drained of excess moisture

seasonings:

½ teaspoon onion powder

¼ teaspoon salt

⅛ teaspoon black pepper

You'll need: medium bowl, large skillet, nonstick spray

Prep: 5 minutes
Cook: 5 minutes

Plus prep and cook times for spaghetti squash (pages 241–243) if not made in advance.

1. In a medium bowl, combine all ingredients and seasonings *except* spaghetti squash. Stir until uniform.

2. Bring a large skillet sprayed with nonstick spray to medium-high heat. Add spaghetti squash, and cook and stir until squash is hot, about 2 minutes.

3. Reduce heat to medium low. Add cheese mixture, and cook and stir until cheese has melted and coated squash, about 2 minutes.

MAKES 2 SERVINGS

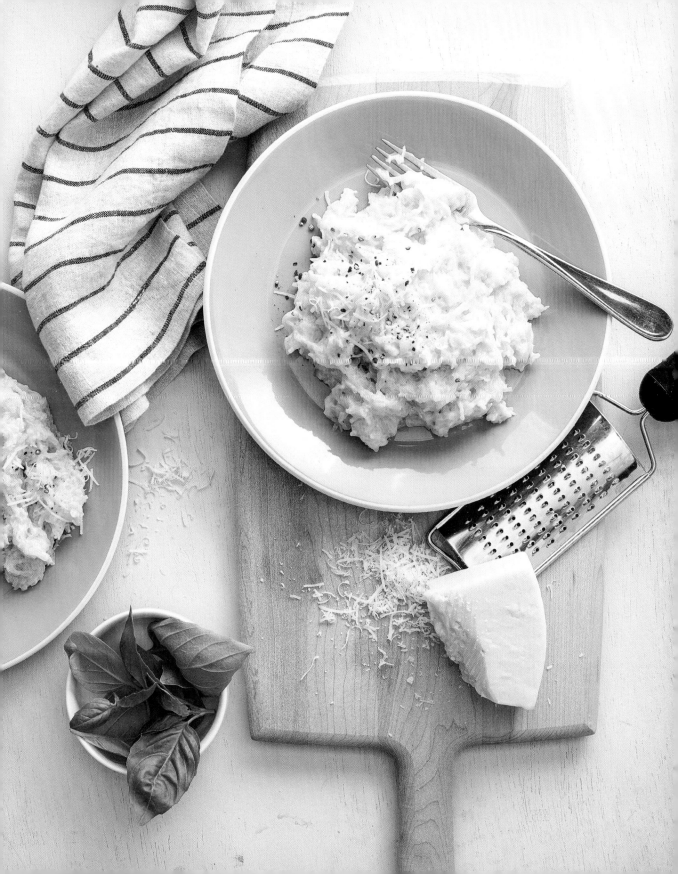

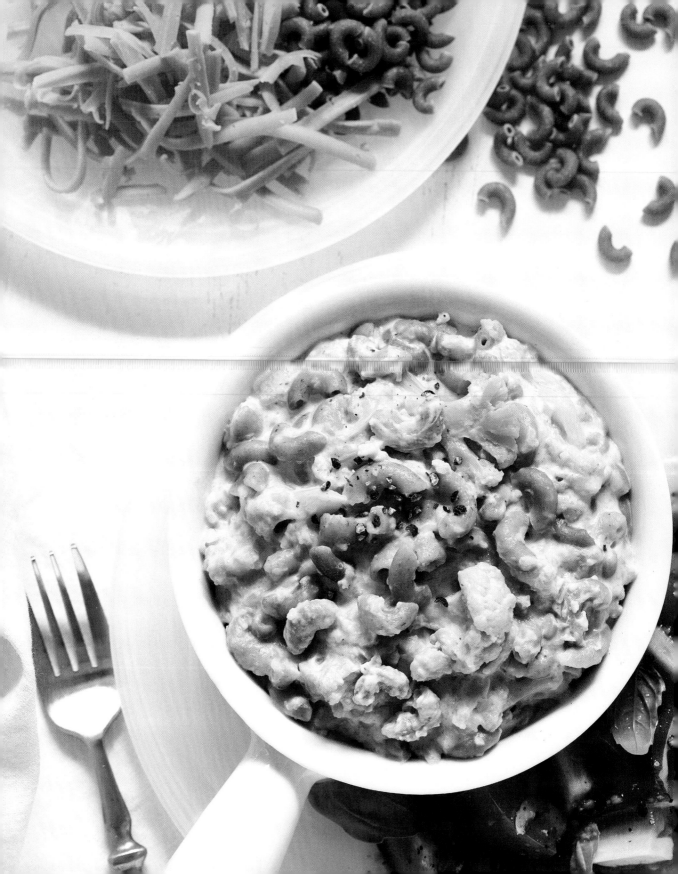

SUPER-SIZED SLOW-COOKER MAC & CHEESE

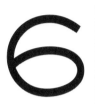 **¼th of recipe (about 1½ cups):** 262 calories, 8g total fat (4g sat fat), 517mg sodium, 39g carbs, 6.5g fiber, 9g sugars, 13g protein

6

5 ounces (about 1½ cups) **uncooked high-fiber elbow macaroni**
6 cups chopped **cauliflower**
½ cup **fat-free milk**
⅓ cup **light/reduced-fat cream cheese**
¼ cup **light sour cream**
¼ cup shredded **reduced-fat cheddar cheese**

seasonings:
1 teaspoon garlic powder
½ teaspoon onion powder
½ teaspoon salt
¼ teaspoon black pepper

You'll need: large pot, slow cooker, nonstick spray, medium microwave-safe bowl

Prep: 10 minutes
Cook: 4 hours 45 minutes

1. In a large pot, cook pasta very al dente, for about half the time indicated on the package. Drain well.

2. Spray a slow cooker with nonstick spray. Add cauliflower and seasonings. Mix well.

3. Add milk, ⅓ cup water, and cooked pasta. Gently stir. Cover and cook on low for about 4½ hours, until cauliflower is tender and pasta is fully cooked.

4. In a medium microwave-safe bowl, stir cream cheese, sour cream, and cheddar until mixed. Microwave for 40 seconds, or until cheeses have melted.

5. Stir cheese mixture until smooth and uniform, and add to the contents of the slow cooker. Stir to coat.

MAKES 4 SERVINGS

WHITE PITA PIZZA

  Entire recipe: 284 calories, 9g total fat (5g sat fat), 748mg sodium, 36g carbs, 7g fiber, 5.5g sugars, 21g protein

¼ cup **light/low-fat ricotta cheese**
1 teaspoon chopped **garlic**
1 **whole-wheat pita**
¼ cup shredded **part-skim mozzarella cheese**
3 **cherry tomatoes**, halved
1 tablespoon chopped **fresh basil**

seasonings:
¼ teaspoon Italian seasoning
¼ teaspoon onion powder
Dash each salt and black pepper

284 CALORIES

You'll need: baking sheet, nonstick spray, small bowl

Prep: 5 minutes
Cook: 15 minutes

1. Preheat oven to 375 degrees. Spray a baking sheet with nonstick spray.

2. In a small bowl, mix ricotta, garlic, and seasonings.

3. Lay pita on the baking sheet and spread with seasoned ricotta, leaving a ½-inch border.

4. Sprinkle with mozzarella. Top with halved cherry tomatoes.

5. Bake until hot and lightly browned, 10 to 12 minutes.

6. Top with basil.

MAKES 1 SERVING

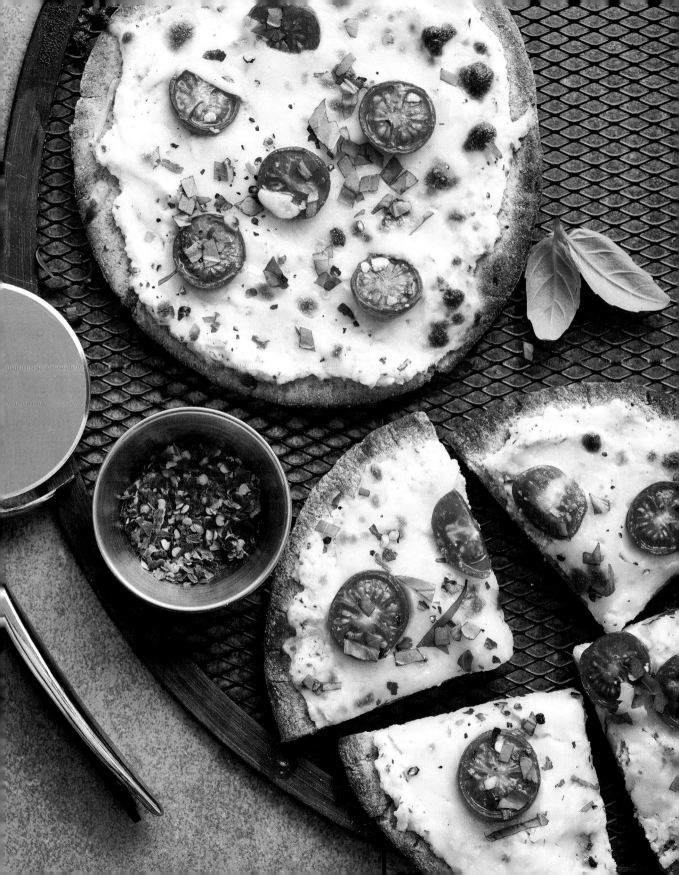

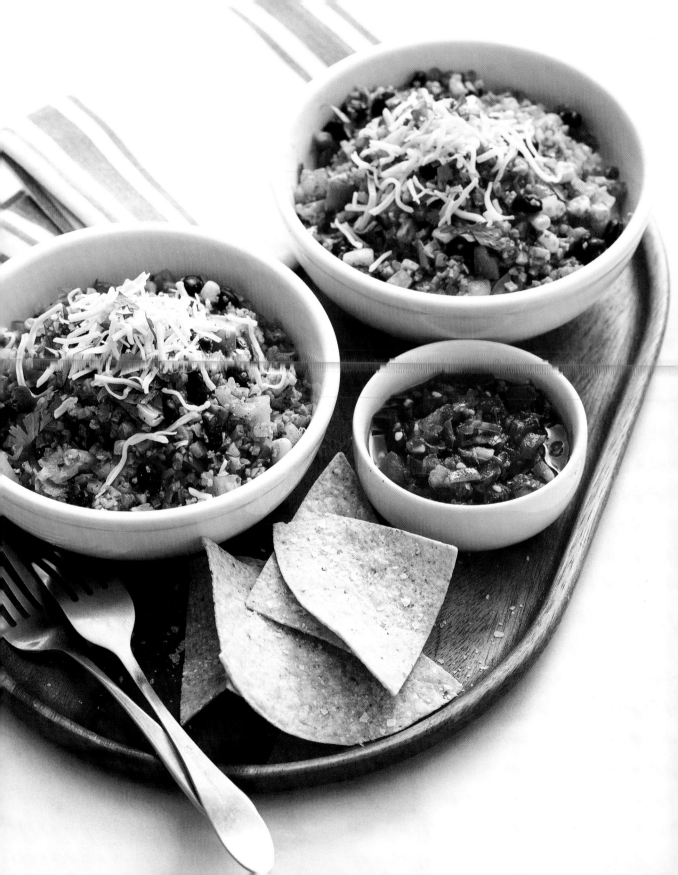

MEXICAN CAULIFLOWER RICE

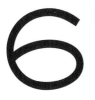 **¼th of recipe (about ¾ cup):** 149 calories, 3.5g total fat (2g sat fat), 498mg sodium, 22.5g carbs, 5.5g fiber, 5.5g sugars, 9g protein

6

½ cup **frozen sweet corn kernels**
4 cups **riced cauliflower**
½ cup chopped **green bell pepper**
½ cup chopped **onion**
½ cup **canned black beans**, drained and rinsed
½ cup shredded **reduced-fat Mexican blend cheese**

seasonings:
2½ tablespoons taco seasoning

149
CALORIES

You'll need: extra-large skillet, nonstick spray, bowl

Prep: 5 minutes
Cook: 15 minutes

1. Bring an extra-large skillet sprayed with nonstick spray to medium-high heat. Cook and stir corn until blackened, about 5 minutes. Transfer to a bowl.

2. Remove skillet from heat; clean, if needed. Respray, and return to medium-high heat. Add cauliflower, pepper, onion, taco seasoning, and 1 tablespoon water. Cook and stir until veggies have mostly softened, 6 to 8 minutes.

3. Add beans and blackened corn, and cook and stir until hot and well mixed, about 1 minute.

4. Serve topped with cheese.

MAKES 4 SERVINGS

HG FYI

Everything you need to know about riced cauliflower is on page 365!

MUSHROOM FAUX-SOTTO

 ¼th of recipe (about ¾ cup): 132 calories, 6g total fat (3.5g sat fat), 524mg sodium, 14.5g carbs, 4g fiber, 6g sugars, 8g protein

6

2 cups thinly sliced **brown mushrooms**
1 cup diced **onion**
2 teaspoons chopped **garlic**
4 cups **riced cauliflower**
⅓ cup **light/reduced-fat cream cheese**
2 tablespoons plus 2 teaspoons grated **Parmesan cheese**

seasonings:
½ teaspoon salt
¼ teaspoon black pepper

132 CALORIES

You'll need: extra-large skillet with lid, nonstick spray, medium bowl

Prep: 10 minutes
Cook: 15 minutes

1. Bring an extra-large skillet sprayed with nonstick spray to medium-high heat. Add mushrooms, onion, and garlic. Cook and stir until browned, about 3 minutes.

2. Add cauliflower and ¼ cup water. Cover and cook for 6 minutes.

3. Meanwhile, in a medium bowl, combine cream cheese, 2 tablespoons Parm, and seasonings. Mix until uniform.

4. Uncover skillet. Cook and stir until water has evaporated and veggies are tender, about 2 minutes.

5. Reduce heat to medium low. Add cream cheese mixture, and cook and stir until mixture has melted and coated the veggies, about 1 minute.

6. Serve topped with remaining 2 teaspoons Parm.

MAKES 4 SERVINGS

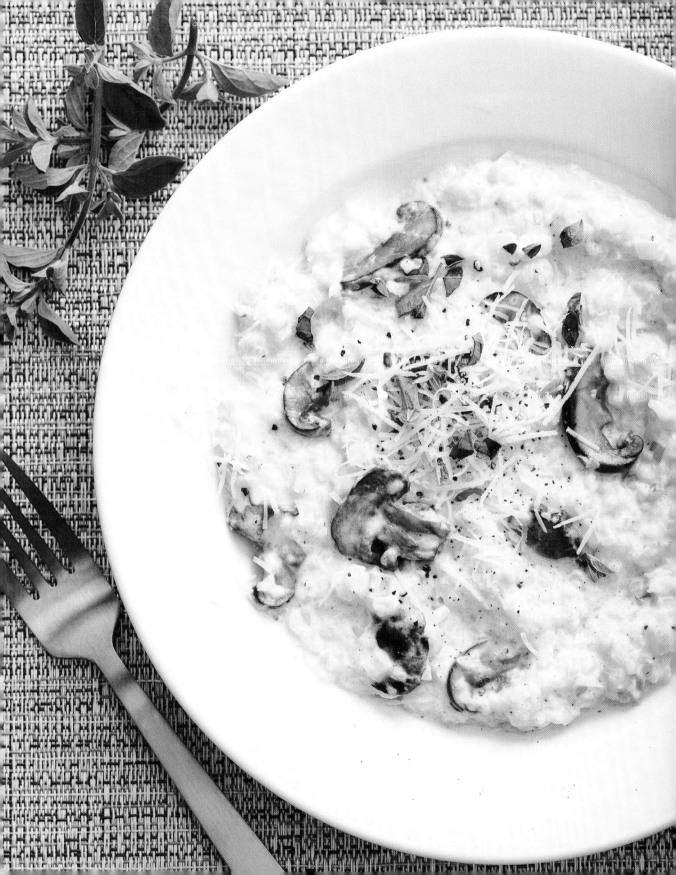

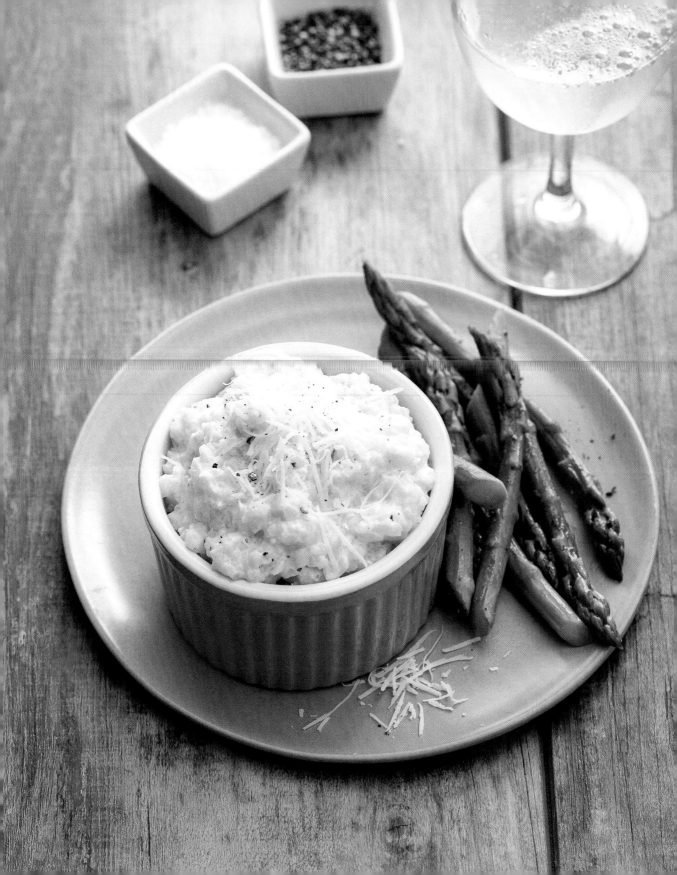

CHEESY FAUX-SOTTO

 ¼th of recipe (about ⅔ cup): 139 calories, 9g total fat (5.5g sat fat), 544mg sodium, 9.5g carbs, 3g fiber, 3.5g sugars, 6.5g protein

5

⅓ cup **light/reduced-fat cream cheese**
2 tablespoons plus 2 teaspoons grated **Parmesan cheese**
2 tablespoons **whipped butter**
2 teaspoons chopped **garlic**
3¾ cups **riced cauliflower**

seasonings:
1 teaspoon onion powder
½ teaspoon salt
¼ teaspoon black pepper

You'll need: medium bowl, extra-large skillet with lid, nonstick spray

Prep: 10 minutes
Cook: 10 minutes

1. In a medium bowl, combine cream cheese, 2 tablespoons Parm, butter, garlic, and seasonings. Stir until mostly smooth and uniform.

2. Bring an extra-large skillet sprayed with nonstick spray to medium-high heat. Add cauliflower and ¼ cup water. Cover and cook for 6 minutes.

3. Uncover skillet. Cook and stir until cauliflower is tender and water has evaporated, about 2 minutes.

4. Reduce heat to medium low. Add cream cheese mixture, and cook and stir until melted and well mixed, about 1 minute.

5. Serve topped with remaining 2 teaspoons Parm.

MAKES 4 SERVINGS

SUPER-SIZED POTATO SALAD

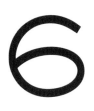

⅕th of recipe (about 1 cup): 166 calories, 6.5g total fat (1g sat fat), 626mg sodium, 21.5g carbs, 4g fiber, 6.5g sugars, 5.5g protein

6

4 cups roughly chopped **cauliflower** (about 1 medium head)
½ cup **light mayonnaise**
½ cup **fat-free plain Greek yogurt**
2 tablespoons **seasoned rice vinegar**
12 ounces (about 2 medium) **white potatoes** cut into bite-sized pieces
1 cup chopped **celery**

seasonings:
½ teaspoon garlic powder
½ teaspoon onion powder
½ teaspoon salt
½ teaspoon dried dill

166 CALORIES

You'll need: large microwave-safe bowl, blender or food processor

Prep: 15 minutes
Cook: 15 minutes
Chill: 1 hour

1. Place 2 cups cauliflower in a large microwave-safe bowl. Add ¼ cup water. Cover and microwave for 6 minutes.

2. Once cool enough to handle, drain well, and transfer to a blender or food processor. Add mayo, yogurt, vinegar, garlic powder, onion powder, salt, and 1 tablespoon water. Blend/process until smooth and uniform.

3. Place potatoes and remaining 2 cups cauliflower in the large bowl. Add ¼ cup water. Cover and microwave for 6 minutes.

4. Once cool enough to handle, drain well, and return to the large bowl. Add blended cauliflower mixture, and stir to coat.

5. Stir in celery and dried dill. Cover and refrigerate until chilled, at least 1 hour.

MAKES 5 SERVINGS

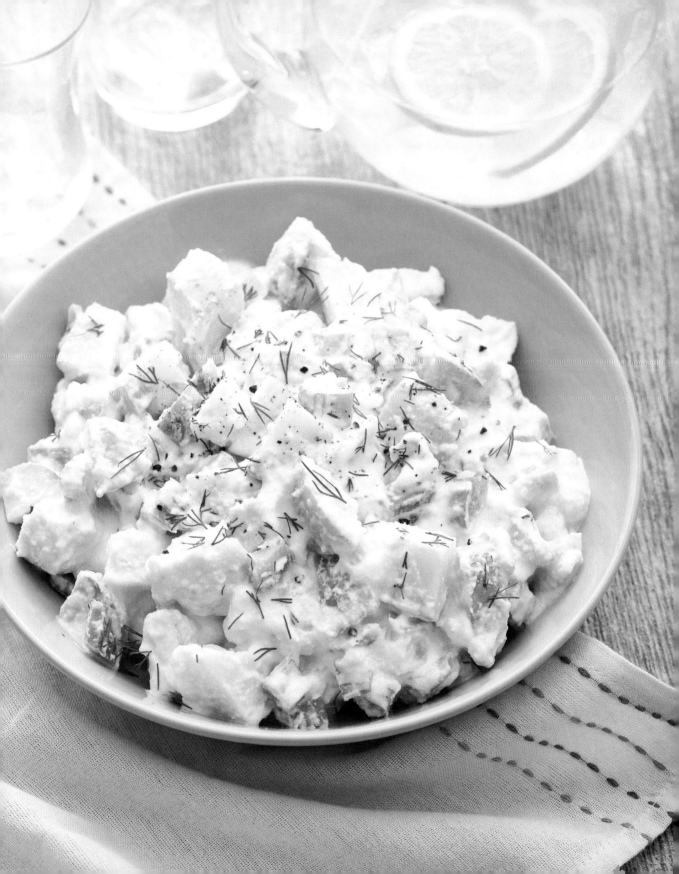

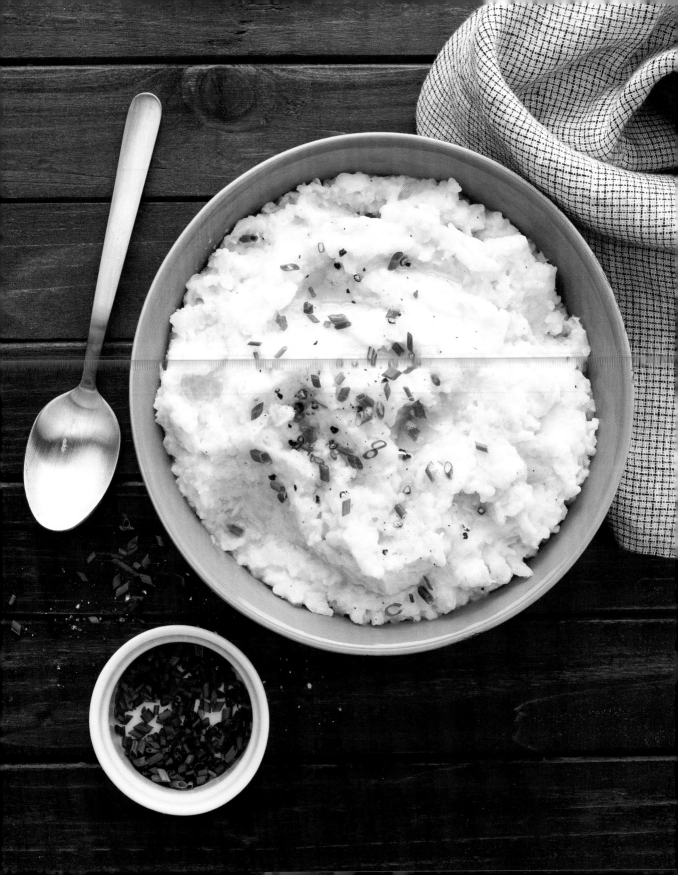

SIMPLE MASHIES

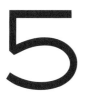 **⅙th of recipe (about ⅔ cup):** 105 calories, 4g total fat (2g sat fat), 188mg sodium, 15g carbs, 3.5g fiber, 3g sugars, 3.5g protein

5

6 cups **cauliflower florets** (about 1 large head)
12 ounces (about 2 medium) **white potatoes**, peeled and cubed
3 tablespoons **light/reduced-fat cream cheese**
2 tablespoons **whipped butter**
2 tablespoons chopped **chives**

seasonings:
½ teaspoon garlic powder
¼ teaspoon salt
⅛ teaspoon black pepper

105 CALORIES

You'll need: large pot, large bowl, potato masher

Prep: 10 minutes
Cook: 35 minutes

1. Bring a large pot of water to a boil.

2. Add cauliflower and potato. Once returned to a boil, reduce heat to medium. Cook until very tender, 15 to 20 minutes.

3. Drain and transfer to a large bowl. Add remaining ingredients *except* chives, and thoroughly mash and mix.

4. Top with chives.

MAKES 6 SERVINGS

BEST BUTTERNUT FRIES

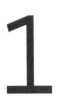 **½ of recipe:** 204 calories, 0.5g total fat (0g sat fat), 309mg sodium, 53g carbs, 9g fiber, 10g sugars, 4.5g protein

1

One 2-pound or half of a 4-pound **butternut squash**, peeled and seeded

seasonings:
¼ teaspoon each salt and black pepper

You'll need:
2 baking sheets, nonstick spray, vegetable peeler (or knife)

Prep: 15 minutes
Cook: 40 minutes

1. Preheat oven to 425 degrees. Spray 2 baking sheets with nonstick spray.

2. Cut squash into fry-shaped spears, and evenly place on the sheets.

3. Sprinkle with salt and pepper. Bake until tender on the inside and crispy on the outside, 15 to 20 minutes per side.

MAKES 2 SERVINGS

HG TIPS

- **Choose a long & narrow squash with a short round section. The long portion is ideal for fry-shaped spears, while the round part is full of seeds and slightly more difficult to manage.**

- **If the squash is too firm to easily cut, microwave it for several minutes to soften. Your hand will thank you!**

PERFECT PARSNIP FRIES

V **GF** **½ of recipe:** 128 calories, 0.5g total fat (0g sat fat), 162mg sodium, 30.5g carbs, 8.5g fiber, 8g sugars, 2g protein

1

12 ounces (about 1 medium-large) **parsnip**

seasonings:
⅛ teaspoon each salt and black pepper

128 CALORIES

You'll need: baking sheet, nonstick spray

Prep: 10 minutes
Cook: 25 minutes

1. Preheat oven to 425 degrees. Spray a baking sheet with nonstick spray.

2. Cut parsnip into fry-shaped spears, and place on the baking sheet.

3. Sprinkle with salt and pepper. Bake until tender on the inside and crispy on the outside, 10 to 15 minutes per side.

MAKES 2 SERVINGS

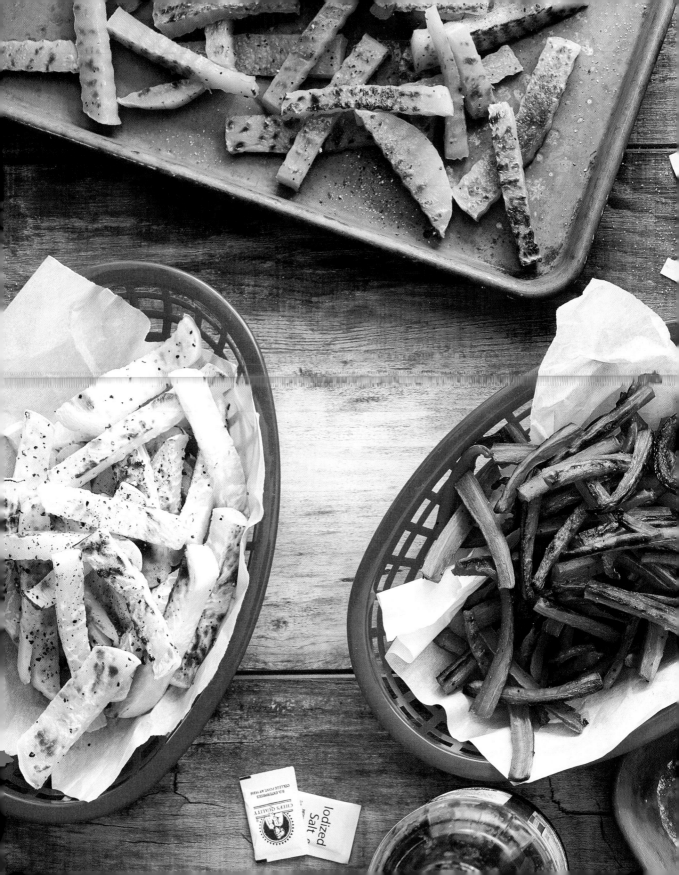

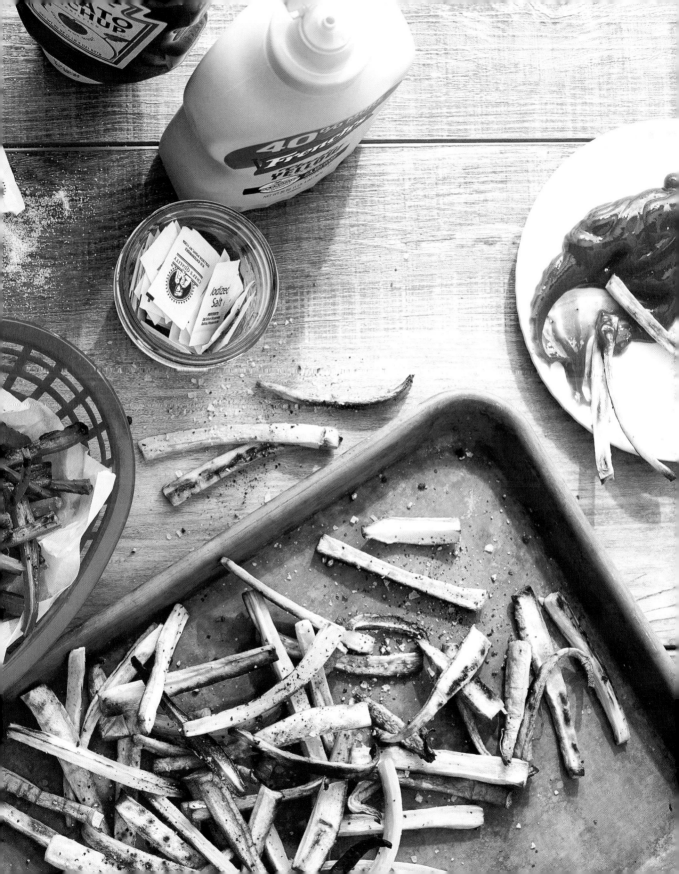

CRISPY CARROT FRIES

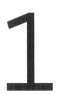 ½ **of recipe:** 139 calories, 0.5g total fat (0g sat fat), 525mg sodium, 32.5g carbs, 9.5g fiber, 16g sugars, 3g protein

1
1½ pounds (about 8 large) **carrots**, peeled

seasonings:
¼ teaspoon each salt and black pepper

139 CALORIES

You'll need:
2 baking sheets, nonstick spray

Prep: 15 minutes
Cook: 30 minutes

1. Preheat oven to 425 degrees. Spray 2 baking sheets with nonstick spray.

2. Cut carrots into fry-shaped spears, and evenly place on the sheets.

3. Sprinkle with salt and pepper. Bake until tender on the inside and crispy on the outside, about 15 minutes per side.

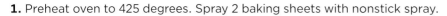

MAKES 2 SERVINGS

TURNIP THE FRIES

 ½ **of recipe:** 96 calories, <0.5g total fat (0g sat fat), 373mg sodium, 22g carbs, 6g fiber, 13g sugars, 3g protein

1
1½ pounds (about 2 medium) **turnips**, peeled

seasonings:
⅛ teaspoon each salt and black pepper

96 CALORIES

You'll need:
2 baking sheets, nonstick spray

Prep: 10 minutes
Cook: 30 minutes

1. Preheat oven to 425 degrees. Spray 2 baking sheets with nonstick spray.

2. Cut turnips into fry-shaped spears, and evenly place on the sheets.

3. Sprinkle with salt and pepper. Bake until tender on the inside and crispy on the outside, about 15 minutes per side.

MAKES 2 SERVINGS

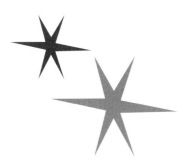

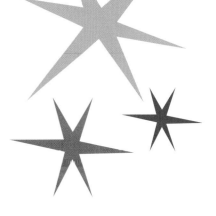

6 Tips for Veggie Fries

1. Size matters. The thicker the fries, the longer the cook time. Cut your fries uniformly so they cook up evenly.

2. Crinkle cut. Get yourself a crinkle cutter (they're totally affordable!) to make authentic-looking French fries.

3. Avoid crowds. If your fries are too close together on the baking sheet, they won't crisp up. When in doubt, use another sheet.

4. Experiment with seasonings. Try cumin and garlic powder, or give cinnamon a go!

5. Dip it good. Reach for ketchup, hot sauce, BBQ sauce, honey mustard . . . the sky's the limit!

6. Need to reheat? Skip the microwave. A toaster oven will give you crispier results!

VEGGIE PIZZA-DILLA

 Entire recipe: 261 calories, 9.5g total fat (5g sat fat), 729mg sodium, 34g carbs, 8.5g fiber, 6g sugars, 17.5g protein

5

¼ cup chopped **bell pepper**
¼ cup chopped **mushrooms**
1 **large high-fiber flour tortilla** with 110 calories or less
⅓ cup shredded **part-skim mozzarella cheese**
⅓ cup **canned crushed tomatoes**

seasonings:
¼ teaspoon Italian seasoning
⅛ teaspoon garlic powder
⅛ teaspoon onion powder

You'll need: skillet, nonstick spray, medium bowl, spatula, small microwave-safe bowl

Prep: 5 minutes
Cook: 10 minutes

1. Bring a skillet sprayed with nonstick spray to medium-high heat. Add pepper, mushrooms, and ⅛ teaspoon Italian seasoning.

2. Cook and stir until softened and lightly browned, about 4 minutes. Transfer to a medium bowl.

3. Remove skillet from heat; clean, if needed. Respray, and bring to medium heat. Add tortilla, and top one half with cheese. Spoon veggies over the other half of the tortilla. Cook until cheese melts, about 2 minutes.

4. Using a spatula, fold the cheese-only tortilla half over the filling, and press lightly to seal. Carefully flip and cook until crispy, about 2 minutes.

5. In a small microwave-safe bowl, mix crushed tomatoes with garlic powder, onion powder, and remaining ⅛ teaspoon Italian seasoning. Cover and microwave for 30 seconds, or until hot.

6. Slice into wedges, and serve with seasoned tomatoes for dipping.

MAKES 1 SERVING

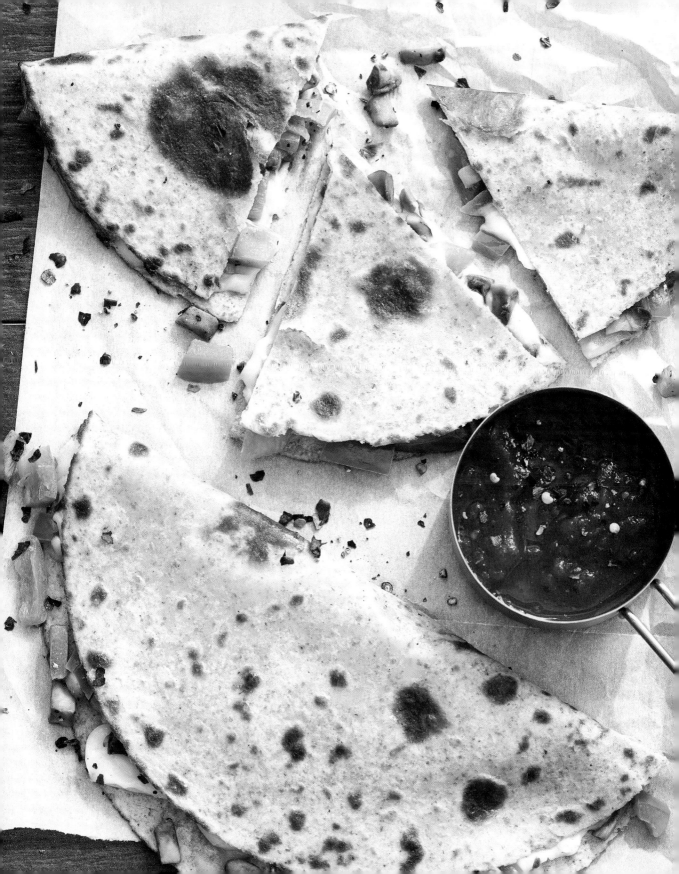

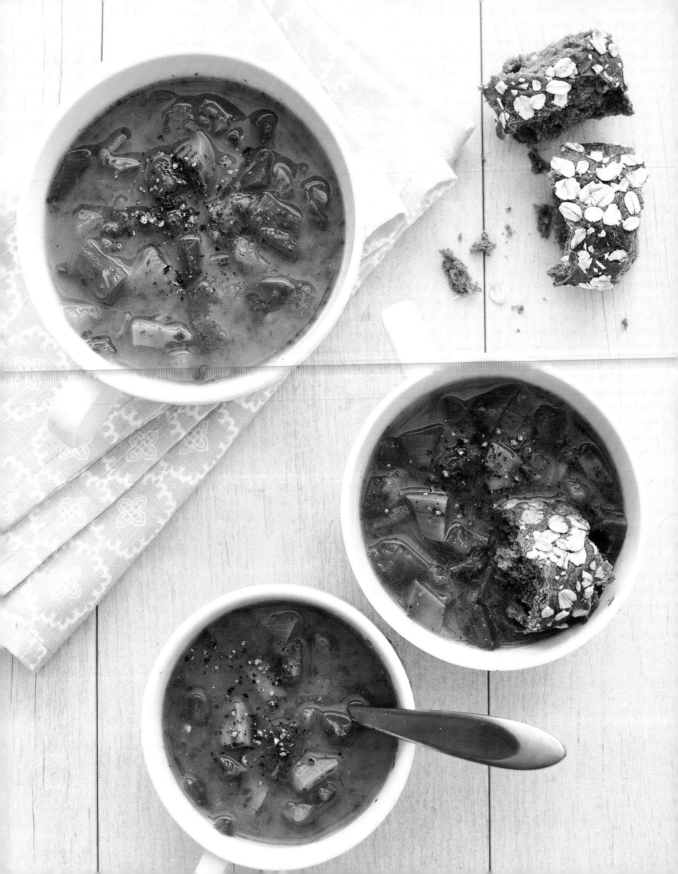

BUTTERNUT 'N KALE SOUP

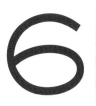 ¹⁄₁₀th of recipe (about 1 cup): 74 calories, 1g total fat (0g sat fat), 487mg sodium, 14.5g carbs, 3g fiber, 5.5g sugars, 2.5g protein

6

8 ounces (about 3 cups) **frozen chopped kale**

4 cups **vegetable broth**

4 cups **creamy butternut squash soup** with 100 calories or less per serving

3 cups chopped **mushrooms**

2 cups chopped **red bell pepper**

1 cup chopped **onion**

seasonings:
2 teaspoons garlic powder
1 teaspoon ground cumin
¼ teaspoon black pepper

74 CALORIES

You'll need: blender, large pot with lid

Prep: 15 minutes
Cook: 45 minutes

1. Place kale in a blender. Add 3 cups broth, and puree until smooth.

2. Transfer blended kale to a large pot. Add butternut squash soup, veggies, seasonings, and remaining cup broth. Bring to a boil.

3. Reduce to a simmer. Cover and cook for 30 minutes, or until veggies are soft.

MAKES 10 SERVINGS

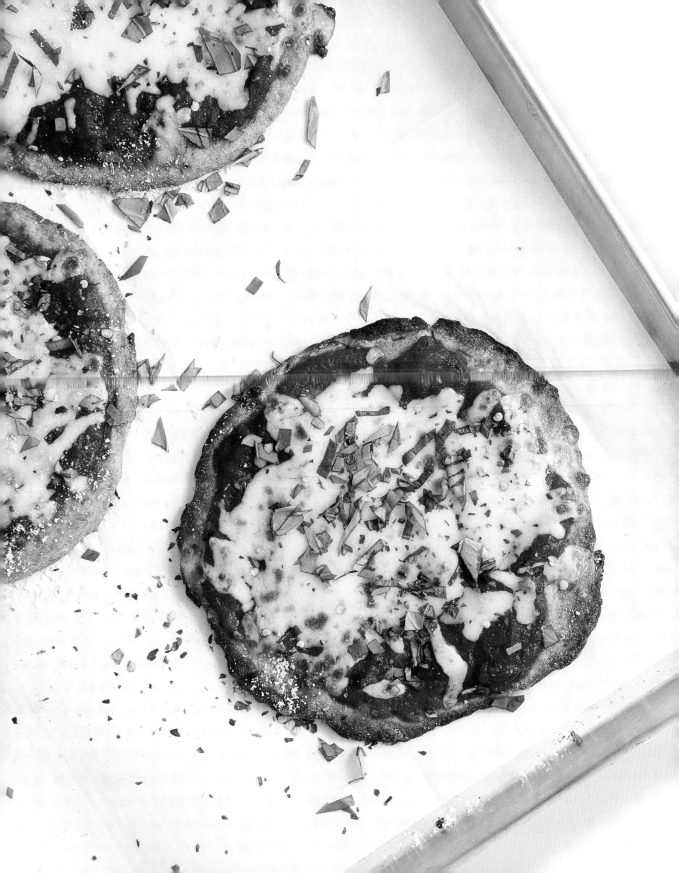

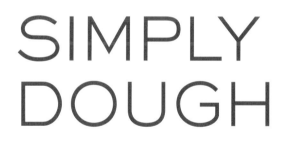

7

SIMPLY DOUGH

My spin on the whole two-ingredient dough trend? A three-ingredient whole-wheat dough made with super-common ingredients! These recipes are game-changing in the best possible way. . .

PIZZA POCKETS

 ½ of recipe (1 pocket): 238 calories, 6g total fat (3g sat fat), 636mg sodium, 29g carbs, 4g fiber, 4.5g sugars, 18g protein

5

½ cup **whole-wheat flour**
¾ teaspoon **baking powder**
½ cup **fat-free plain Greek yogurt**
¼ cup **marinara sauce** with 3g fat or less per serving, or more for dipping
½ cup shredded **part-skim mozzarella cheese**

seasonings:
¼ teaspoon garlic powder
⅛ teaspoon salt

You'll need: baking sheet, nonstick spray, large bowl

Prep: 10 minutes
Cook: 20 minutes

1. Preheat oven to 350 degrees. Spray a baking sheet with nonstick spray.

2. Place flour, baking powder, garlic powder, and salt in a large bowl. Stir until uniform.

3. Add yogurt. Thoroughly mix until a dough-like texture is reached.

4. Evenly form into 2 squares, about 6 inches by 6 inches. Place on the baking sheet, evenly spaced.

5. Evenly spread marinara over bottom half of each square.

6. Sprinkle with cheese.

7. Fold the top half over the mixture so the top edge meets the bottom. Firmly press edges with a fork to seal.

8. Spray with nonstick spray. Bake until tops are light golden brown, about 20 minutes.

MAKES 2 SERVINGS

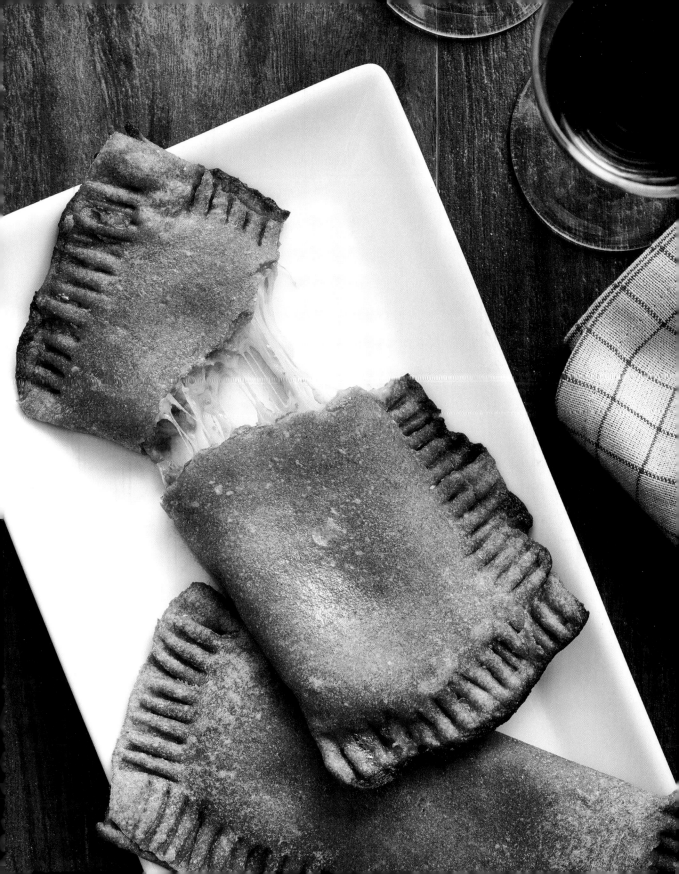

MARGHERITA PIZZA

 ½ of recipe (1 pizza): 241 calories, 6g total fat (3g sat fat), 637mg sodium, 29.5g carbs, 4.5g fiber, 4.5g sugars, 18g protein

6 |
½ cup **whole-wheat flour**
¾ teaspoon **baking powder**
½ cup **fat-free plain Greek yogurt**
¼ cup **marinara sauce** with 3g fat or less per serving
½ cup shredded **part-skim mozzarella cheese**
1 tablespoon chopped **fresh basil**

seasonings:
½ teaspoon garlic powder
¼ teaspoon Italian seasoning
⅛ teaspoon salt

You'll need: baking sheet, parchment paper, large bowl

Prep: 10 minutes
Cook: 15 minutes

1. Preheat oven to 450 degrees. Line a baking sheet with parchment paper.

2. In a large bowl, combine flour, baking powder, and seasonings. Mix until uniform.

3. Add yogurt to the bowl. Thoroughly mix until a dough-like texture is reached.

4. To form the crusts, evenly divide dough into two circles on the parchment-lined baking sheet, each about ⅛-inch thick and 6 inches in diameter.

5. Bake for 7 minutes.

6. Spread sauce over each crust, leaving a ½-inch border. Evenly sprinkle with cheese.

7. Bake until cheese has melted and crust is crispy, about 5 minutes.

8. Top with basil.

MAKES 2 SERVINGS

EXTRA, EXTRA!

There's no wrong way to top a pizza, but I love this one with Parm and red pepper flakes!

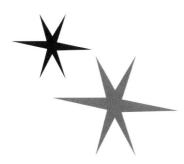

Hungry for More Pizza?

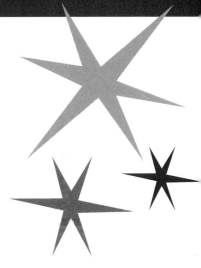

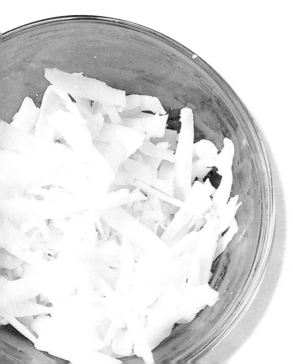

SURVEY SAYS . . .

A whopping 69% of Hungry Girl fans say thin crust is better than thick. Smart humans!

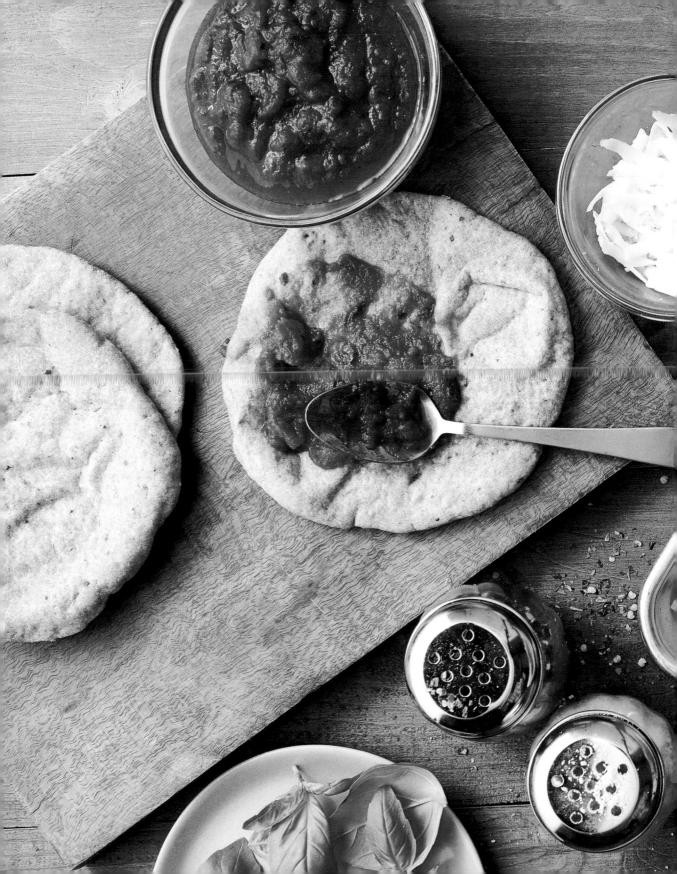

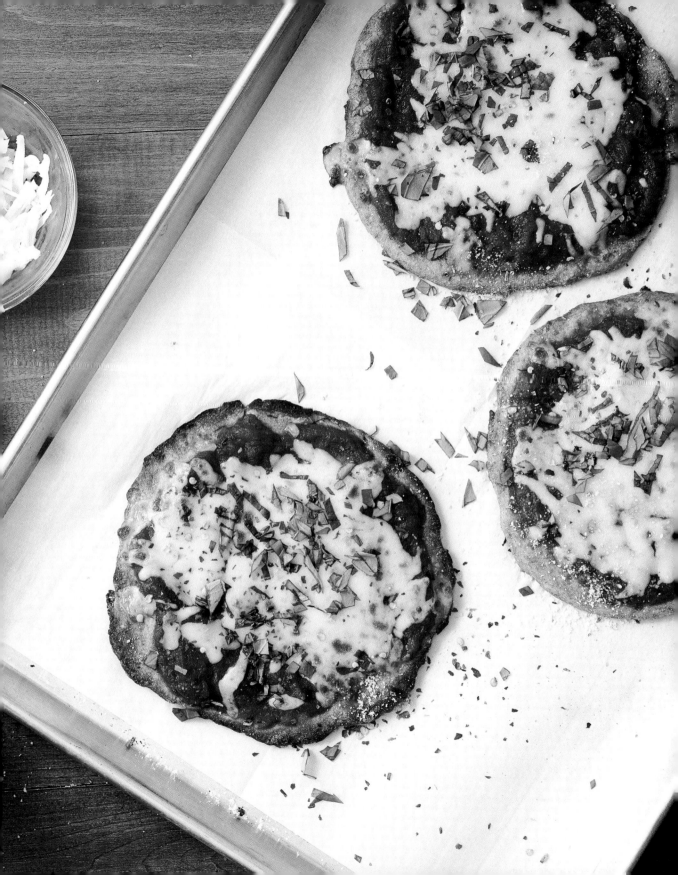

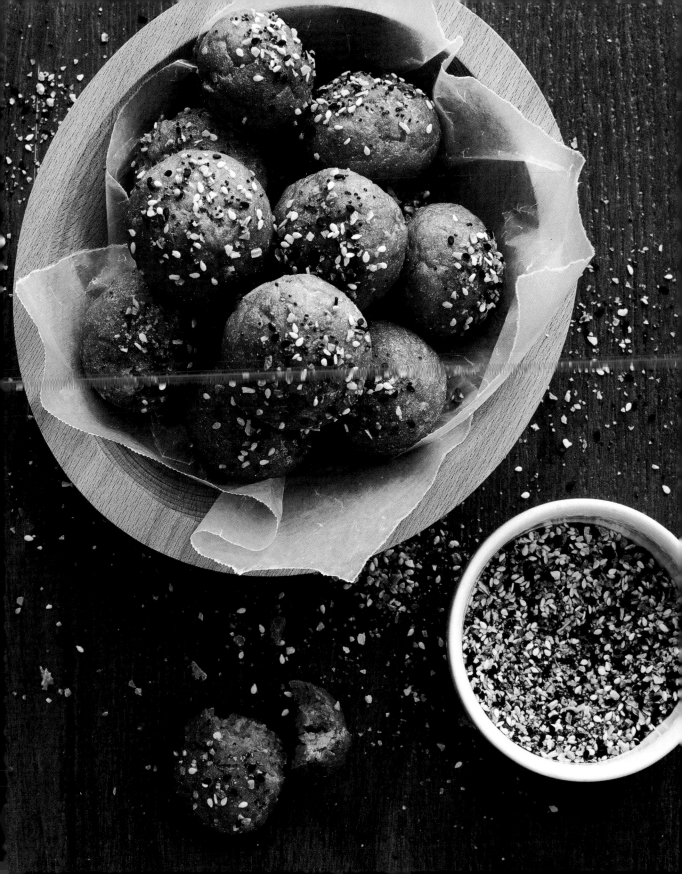

EVERYTHING BAGEL BITES

 ½ of recipe (4 bites): 156 calories, 0.5g total fat (0g sat fat), 529mg sodium, 25.5g carbs, 3.5g fiber, 2.5g sugars, 11g protein

4

½ cup **whole-wheat flour**
¾ teaspoon **baking powder**
½ cup **fat-free plain Greek yogurt**
2 tablespoons (about 1 large) **egg white** or **fat-free liquid egg substitute**

seasonings:
⅛ teaspoon salt
1 teaspoon everything bagel seasoning blend

 156 CALORIES

You'll need: baking sheet, nonstick spray, large bowl, pastry brush (optional)

Prep: 10 minutes
Cook: 15 minutes

1. Preheat oven to 350 degrees. Spray a baking sheet with nonstick spray.

2. Place flour, baking powder, salt, and ½ teaspoon everything bagel seasoning in a large bowl. Stir until uniform.

3. Add yogurt. Thoroughly mix until a dough-like texture is reached.

4. Evenly form into 8 balls (about 2 tablespoons each), and place on the baking sheet, evenly spaced.

5. Brush the tops with egg. Evenly sprinkle with remaining ½ teaspoon everything bagel seasoning.

6. Bake until tops are light golden brown and insides are cooked through, about 15 minutes.

MAKES 2 SERVINGS

HG FYI

DIY seasoning recipe on page 357!

GARLIC KNOTS

30m **V**   **½ of recipe (3 knots):** 192 calories, 5g total fat (2.5g sat fat), 575mg sodium, 26.5g carbs, 4g fiber, 3g sugars, 11g protein

½ cup **whole-wheat flour**
¾ teaspoon **baking powder**
½ cup **fat-free plain Greek yogurt**
1 tablespoon **whipped butter**
½ tablespoon **light/reduced-fat cream cheese**
½ tablespoon grated **Parmesan cheese**

seasonings:
¼ teaspoon salt
¾ teaspoon garlic powder

192 CALORIES

You'll need: baking sheet, nonstick spray, 2 large bowls, rolling pin, medium microwave-safe bowl

Prep: 10 minutes
Cook: 15 minutes

1. Preheat oven to 350 degrees. Spray a baking sheet with nonstick spray.

2. Place flour, baking powder, salt, and ¼ teaspoon garlic powder in a large bowl. Stir until uniform.

3. Add yogurt. Thoroughly mix until a dough-like texture is reached.

4. Roll out dough into a large square of even thickness, about 6 inches by 6 inches. Evenly cut dough into 6 strips, each about 3 inches by 2 inches.

5. Roll and tie each strip into a knot, and place on the baking sheet, evenly spaced.

6. Spray knots with nonstick spray. Bake until tops are light golden brown and insides are cooked through, about 15 minutes.

7. Meanwhile, in a medium microwave-safe bowl, combine butter, cream cheese, and remaining ½ teaspoon garlic powder. Microwave for 20 seconds, or until cream cheese and butter have melted. Whisk with a fork until mostly smooth and uniform.

8. Place rolls in a large bowl. Drizzle with cheese mixture, and toss to coat. Add Parm, and toss to coat again.

MAKES 2 SERVINGS

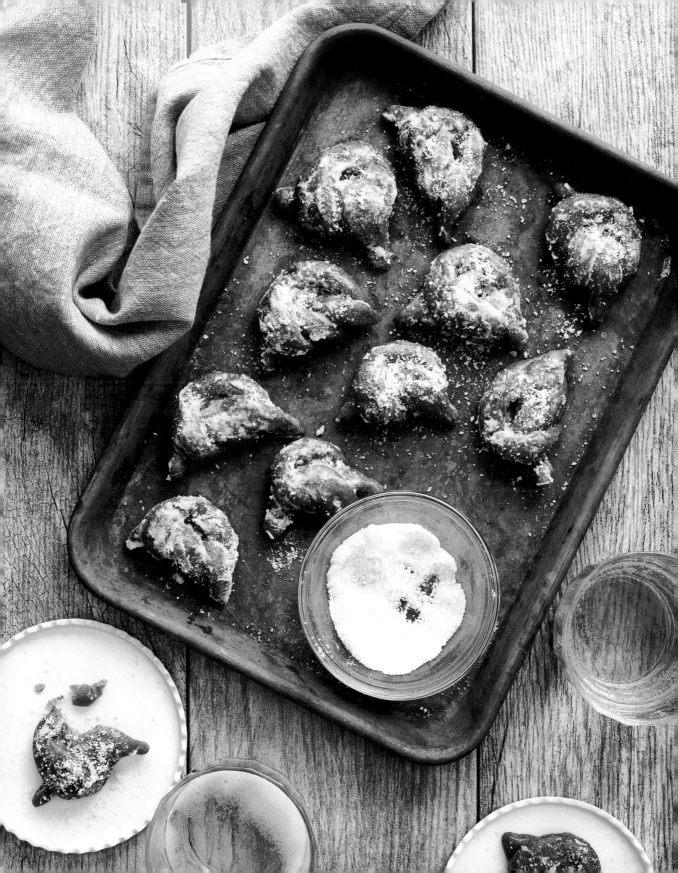

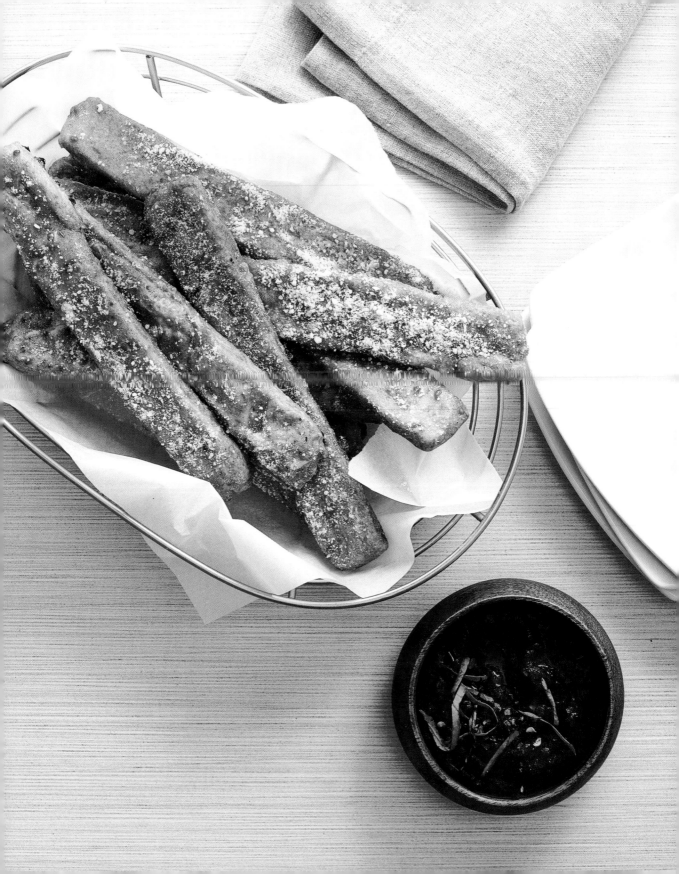

CHEESY BREADSTICKS

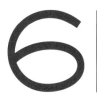 **⅙th of recipe (1 breadstick):** 75 calories, 2g total fat (1g sat fat), 176mg sodium, 8.5g carbs, 1g fiber, 1g sugars, 5g protein

6

½ cup **whole-wheat flour**
¾ teaspoon **baking powder**
½ cup **fat-free plain Greek yogurt**
⅓ cup shredded **part-skim mozzarella cheese**
2 teaspoons **whipped butter**
1½ teaspoons grated **Parmesan cheese**

seasonings:
¼ teaspoon garlic powder
¼ teaspoon Italian seasoning
⅛ teaspoon salt

75 CALORIES

You'll need: baking sheet, nonstick spray, large bowl, medium microwave-safe bowl, pastry brush (optional)

Prep: 10 minutes
Cook: 15 minutes

1. Preheat oven to 350 degrees. Spray a baking sheet with nonstick spray.

2. Place flour, baking powder, and seasonings in a large bowl. Stir until uniform.

3. Add yogurt and mozzarella. Thoroughly mix until a dough-like texture is reached.

4. Roll out dough into a large square of even thickness, about 7 inches by 7 inches. Evenly cut dough into 6 strips, and place on the baking sheet.

5. Bake until tops are light golden brown and insides are cooked through, about 15 minutes.

6. Meanwhile, in a medium microwave-safe bowl, microwave butter 10 seconds, or until melted.

7. Brush the tops with melted butter and sprinkle with Parm.

MAKES 6 SERVINGS

EXTRA, EXTRA!

I love dipping these in marinara . . . Look for sauce with 3 grams of fat or less, or DIY with canned crushed tomatoes and seasonings!

BEAN & CHEESE EMPANADAS

 ½ of recipe (1 empanada): 253 calories, 6.5g total fat (3.5g sat fat), 690mg sodium, 31.5g carbs, 5g fiber, 2.5g sugars, 19g protein

5

½ cup **whole-wheat flour**
¾ teaspoon **baking powder**
½ cup **fat-free plain Greek yogurt**
¼ cup **refried beans**
½ cup shredded **reduced-fat Mexican blend cheese**

seasonings:
⅛ teaspoon salt

253 CALORIES

You'll need: baking sheet, nonstick spray, large bowl

Prep: 10 minutes
Cook: 20 minutes

1. Preheat oven to 350 degrees. Spray a baking sheet with nonstick spray.

2. Place flour, baking powder, and salt in a large bowl. Stir until uniform.

3. Add yogurt. Thoroughly mix until a dough-like texture is reached.

4. Evenly form into 2 circles, about 6 inches in diameter. Place on the baking sheet, evenly spaced.

5. Evenly spread refried beans over one half of each circle.

6. Sprinkle with cheese.

7. Fold the top half over the mixture so the top edge meets the bottom. Firmly press edges with a fork to seal.

8. Spray with nonstick spray. Bake until tops are light golden brown, about 20 minutes.

MAKES 2 SERVINGS

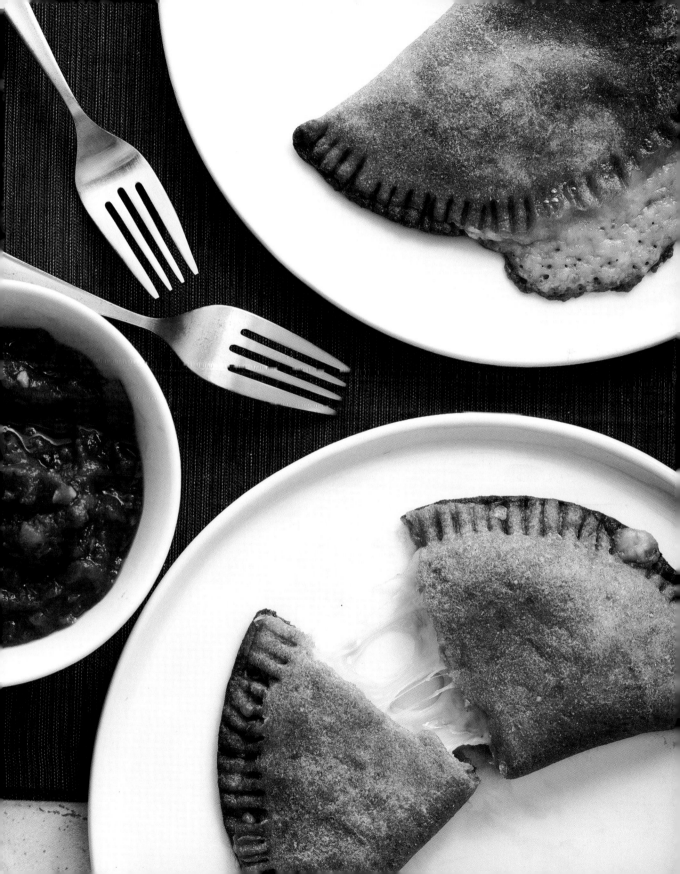

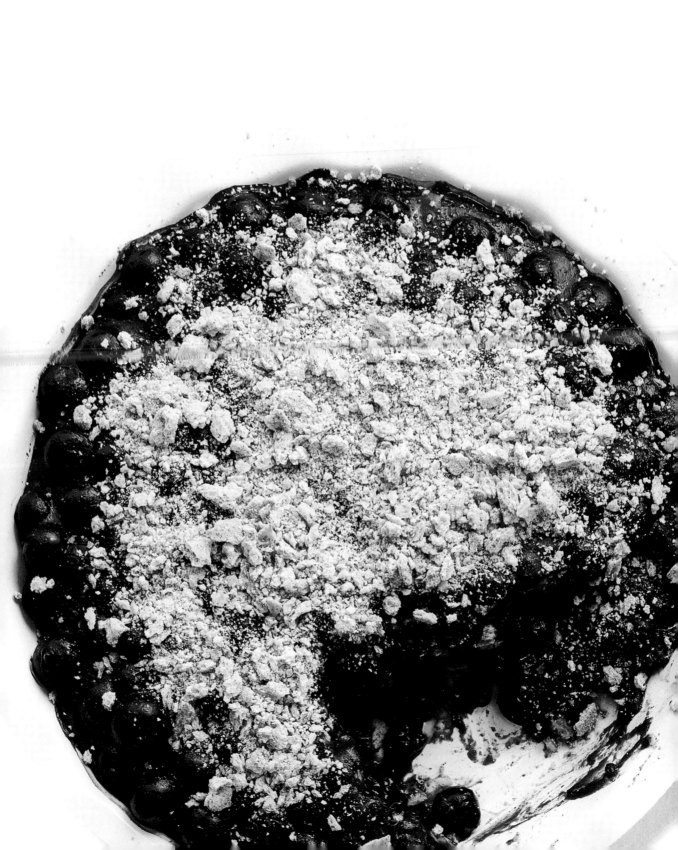

8

SIMPLY FRUIT

Things are about to get sweet! I'm talking breakfast smoothies, slow-cooker pie, the BEST ways to eat an apple, a delicious marriage of blintzes & quesadillas, and more . . .

STRAWBERRY SUPER SMOOTHIE

 Entire recipe: 191 calories, 4g total fat (0.5g sat fat), 257mg sodium, 30.5g carbs, 6.5g fiber, 13.5g sugars, 13.5g protein

6

2 cups **spinach**
1 cup **frozen strawberries** (no sugar added)
1 cup **unsweetened vanilla almond milk**
⅓ cup (about ½ medium) sliced and frozen **banana**
3 tablespoons **vanilla protein powder**
½ cup **crushed ice** (about 3 ice cubes)

191 CALORIES

You'll need: blender

Prep: 5 minutes

1. Place all ingredients in a blender. Add ¼ cup water.

2. Blend until smooth, stopping and stirring if needed.

MAKES 1 SERVING

PROTEIN POWDER 411!

Look for protein powder that has about 100 calories per serving, usually about 1 ounce or 1 full scoop. That serving is equal to about ⅓ cup, but you'll only need a few tablespoons for these recipes!

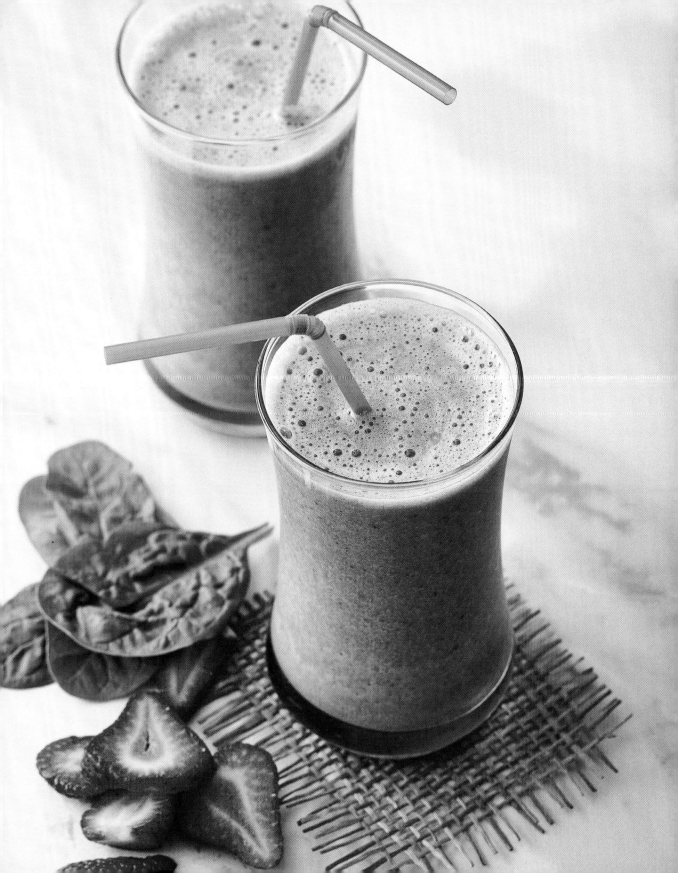

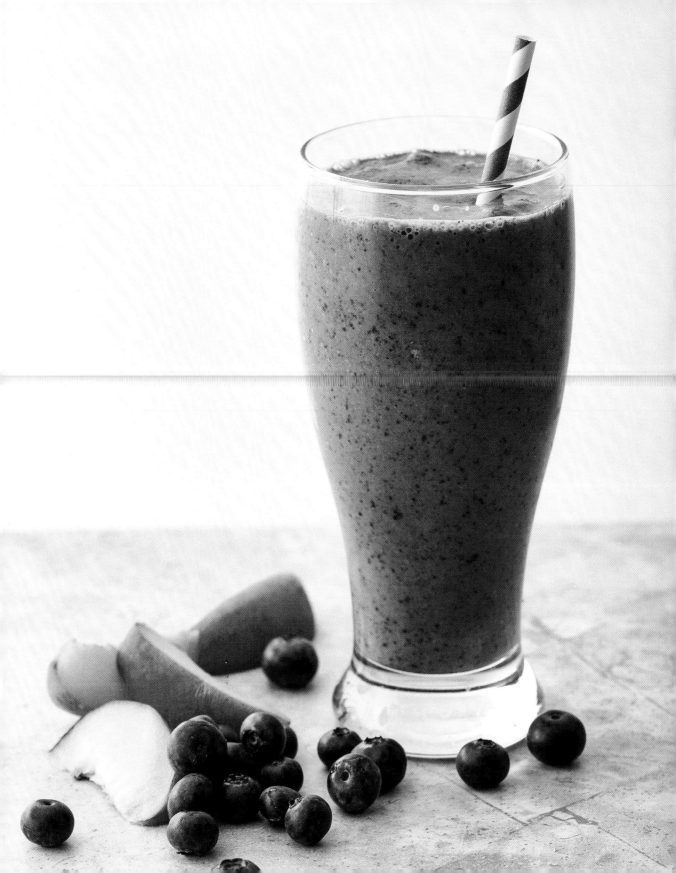

PEACH-BERRY POWER SMOOTHIE

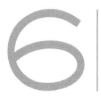 **Entire recipe:** 230 calories, 3g total fat (0g sat fat), 242mg sodium, 34g carbs, 4.5g fiber, 25.5g sugars, 18.5g protein

6

1 cup **frozen peach slices** (no sugar added)
1 cup **unsweetened vanilla almond milk**
⅔ cup **fat-free plain Greek yogurt**
½ cup frozen **blueberries** (no sugar added)
1 packet **natural no-calorie sweetener**
½ cup **crushed ice** (about 3 ice cubes)

230 CALORIES

You'll need: blender

Prep: 5 minutes

1. Place all ingredients in a blender.

2. Blend until smooth and uniform, stopping and stirring if needed.

MAKES 1 SERVING

ORANGE SUNRISE SMOOTHIE

 Entire recipe: 194 calories, 2.5g total fat (0.5g sat fat), 119mg sodium, 36g carbs, 5g fiber, 24.5g sugars, 11.5g protein

6

½ medium **orange** (about ½ cup segments plus zest)
½ cup **unsweetened vanilla almond milk**
⅓ cup **frozen mango chunks**
⅓ cup (about ½ medium) sliced and frozen **banana**
3 tablespoons **vanilla protein powder**
¾ cup **crushed ice** (about 4 ice cubes)

You'll need: fine grater or zester, blender

Prep: 5 minutes

1. Add ½ teaspoon orange zest to a blender.

2. Peel orange, separate into segments, and add to the blender.

3. Add all remaining ingredients. Blend until smooth, stopping and stirring if needed.

MAKES 1 SERVING

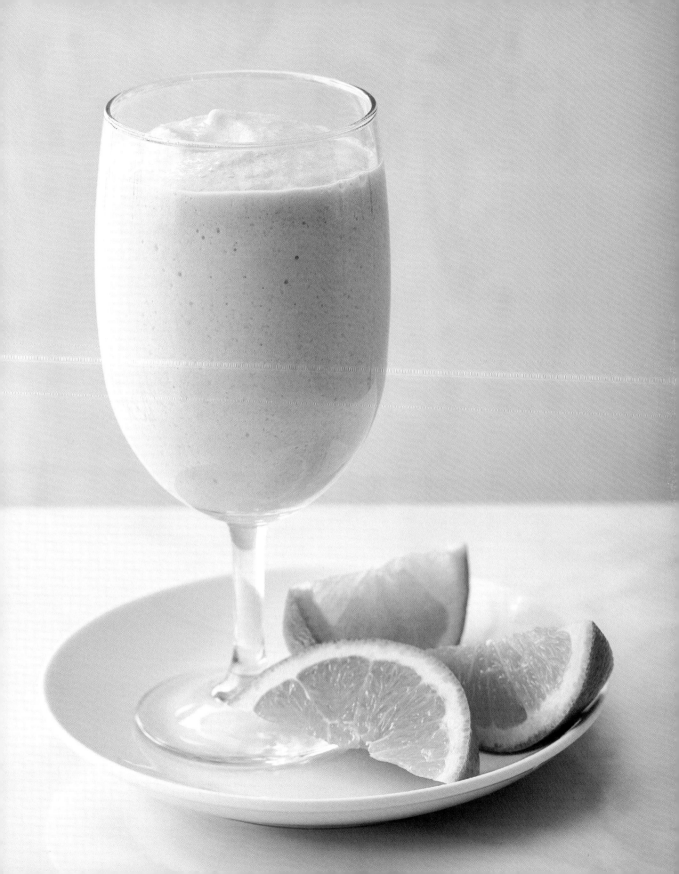

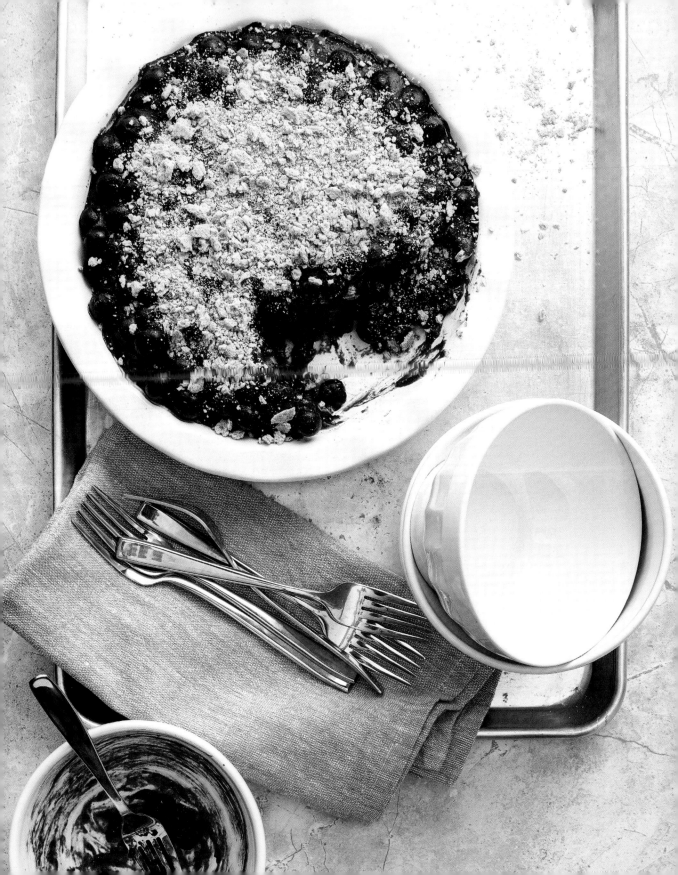

SCOOPABLE UPSIDE-DOWN BLUEBERRY PIE

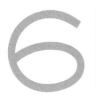

⅛th of recipe: 85 calories, 0.5g total fat (0g sat fat), 94mg sodium, 22.5g carbs, 2.5g fiber, 10.5g sugars, 1g protein

3 tablespoons **cornstarch**
5 cups **blueberries** (fresh or thawed from frozen; no sugar added)
2 tablespoons **Truvia spoonable no-calorie sweetener**
2 teaspoons **lemon juice**
1½ teaspoons **vanilla extract**
2 sheets (8 crackers) **graham crackers**, finely crushed

seasonings:
1½ teaspoons cinnamon
¼ teaspoon nutmeg
¼ teaspoon salt

You'll need: 9-inch deep-dish pie pan, nonstick spray, large nonstick pot

Prep: 5 minutes
Cook: 10 minutes
Cool: 1 hour
Chill: 4 hours

1. Spray a 9-inch deep-dish pie pan with nonstick spray.

2. In a large nonstick pot, combine cornstarch with 1 cup cold water. Stir to dissolve. Add all remaining ingredients and seasonings, *except* graham crackers. Mix well.

3. Set heat to medium. Stirring frequently, cook until thick and gooey, 8 to 10 minutes.

4. Transfer mixture to the pie pan. Let cool completely, about 1 hour.

5. Refrigerate until firm and chilled, at least 4 hours.

6. Just before serving, sprinkle with crushed graham crackers.

MAKES 8 SERVINGS

UPSIDE-DOWN SLOW-COOKER APPLE PIE

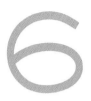 **⅛th of recipe (about ¾ cup):** 80 calories, 0.5g total fat (0g sat fat), 96mg sodium, 23.5g carbs, 2g fiber, 12g sugars, 0.5g protein

8 cups (about 8 medium) peeled and sliced **Granny Smith apples**
2 tablespoons **cornstarch**
3 tablespoons **Truvia spoonable no-calorie sweetener**
2 teaspoons **lemon juice**
1 teaspoon **vanilla extract**
2 sheets (8 crackers) **graham crackers**, finely crushed

seasonings:
1½ teaspoons cinnamon
¼ teaspoon ground nutmeg
¼ teaspoon salt

80 CALORIES

You'll need: slow cooker, nonstick spray, medium bowl

Prep: 5 minutes
Cook: 1½ hours
Cool: 10 minutes

1. Place apples in a slow cooker sprayed with nonstick spray.

2. In a medium bowl, combine cornstarch with ¾ cup water. Whisk with a fork to dissolve. Add all remaining ingredients and seasonings *except* graham crackers. Whisk well.

3. Pour cornstarch mixture over apples, and stir to coat.

4. Cover and cook on high for 1½ hours, or until apples have softened and liquid has mostly thickened.

5. Let cool and thicken, about 10 minutes.

6. Top each serving with 1 crushed graham cracker.

MAKES 8 SERVINGS

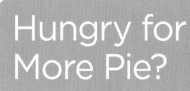

Hungry for More Pie?

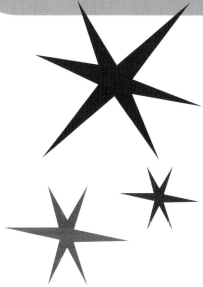

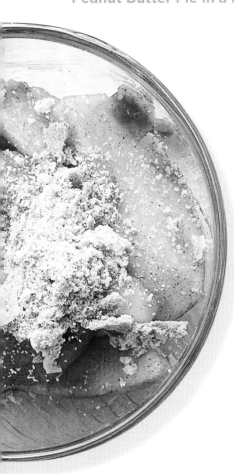

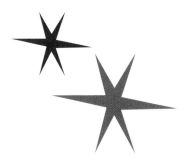

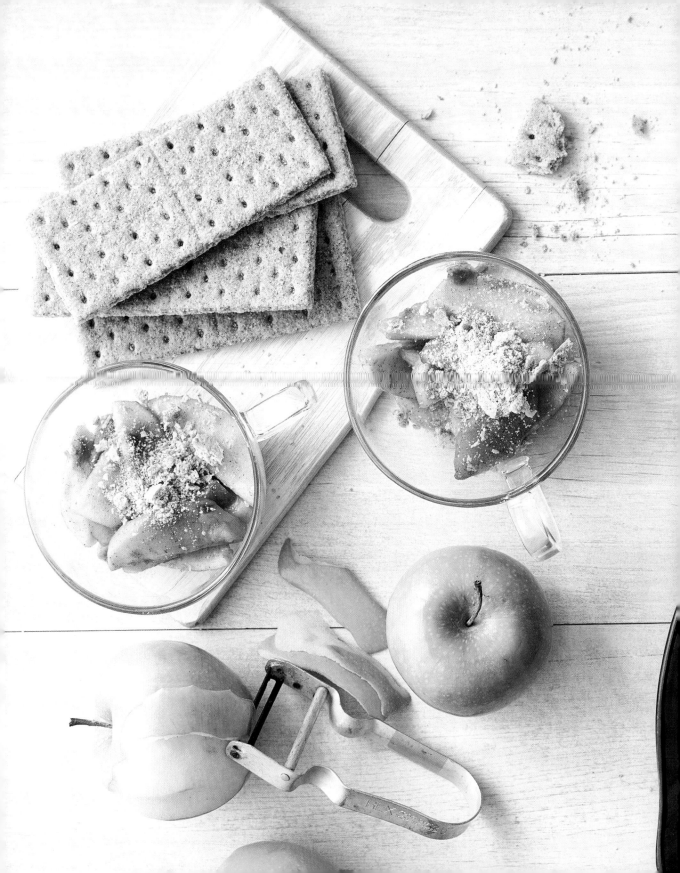

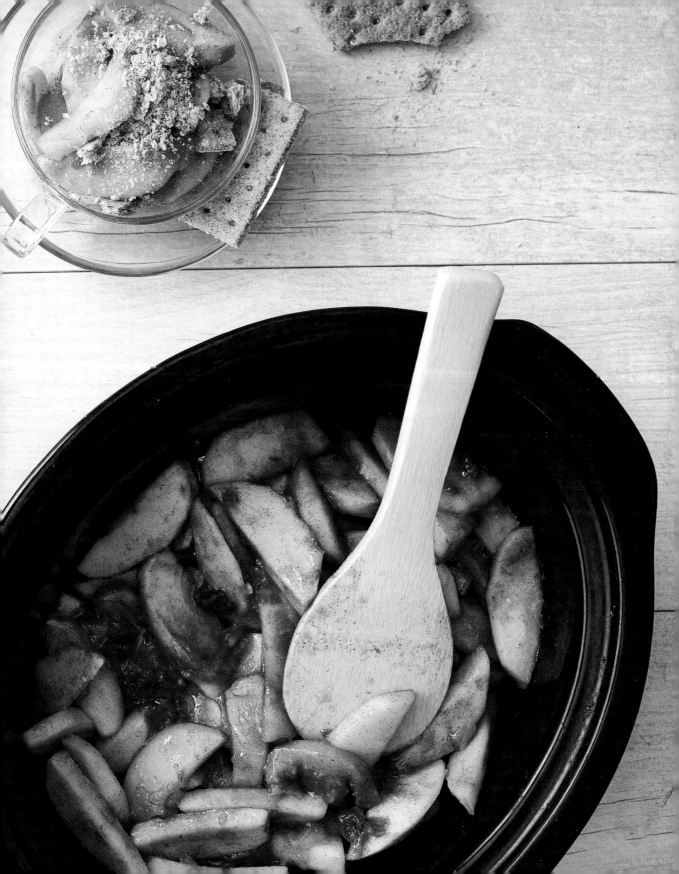

OPEN-FACED APPLE S'MORES

 Entire recipe: 126 calories, 3g total fat (2g sat fat), 28mg sodium, 25.5g carbs, 2.5g fiber, 18.5g sugars, 1g protein

2 teaspoons **mini semi-sweet chocolate chips**
Two round ½-inch-thick **Gala or Fuji apple** slices, cored
2 tablespoons **mini marshmallows**
1 **graham cracker** (¼ sheet), finely crushed

You'll need: small microwave-safe bowl, microwave-safe plate, kitchen torch (optional)

Prep: 5 minutes
Cook: 5 minutes or less

1. In a small microwave-safe bowl, microwave chocolate chips at 50 percent power for 25 seconds. Stir until smooth and uniform.

2. Place apple slices on a microwave-safe plate. Spread chocolate over apple slices. Top with marshmallows.

3. Using a kitchen torch, heat marshmallows until slightly melted and toasted, 5 to 10 seconds. Alternatively, microwave for about 20 seconds.

4. Sprinkle with crushed graham cracker.

MAKES 1 SERVING

HG TIP

Multiply this recipe for a crowd! Your friends will be begging for *s'more* . . .

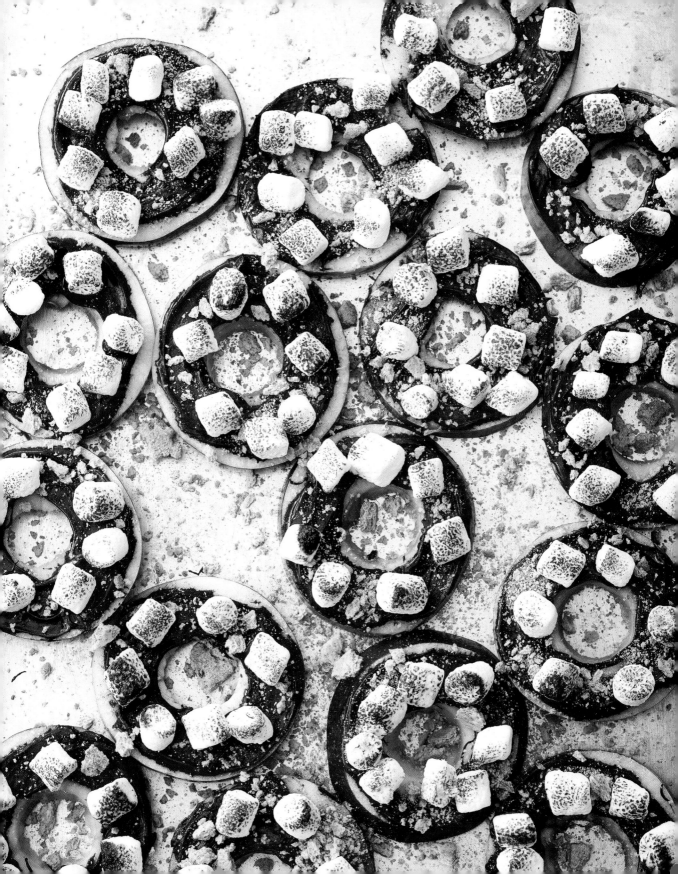

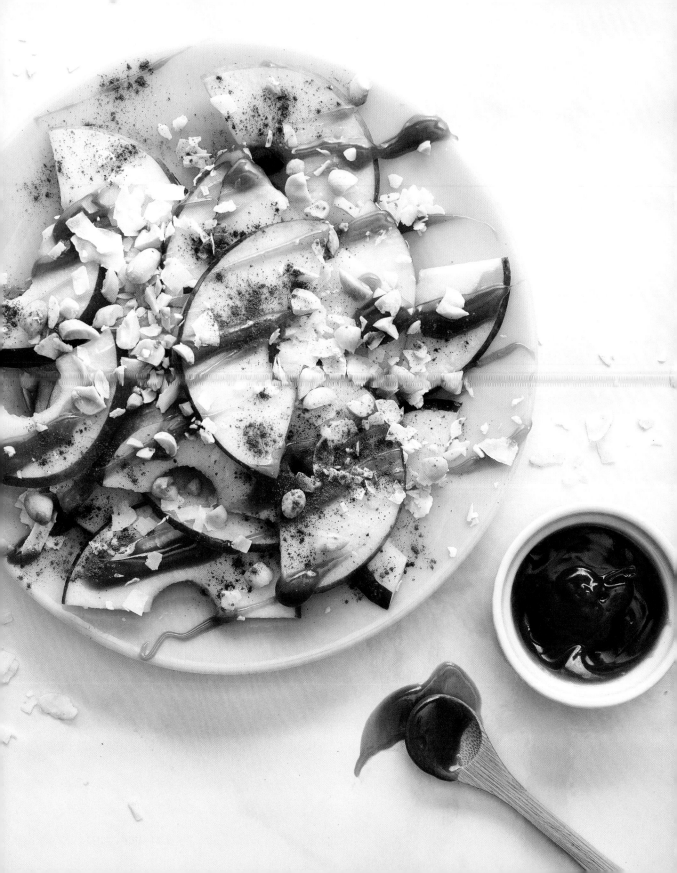

CARAMEL APPLE NACHOS

 ½ of recipe: 171 calories, 3g total fat (0.5g sat fat), 97mg sodium, 37.5g carbs, 3.5g fiber, 25.5g sugars, 2g protein

4

1 large (or 2 small) Gala or Fuji apple(s)
3 tablespoons light caramel dip, room temperature
¼ ounce (about 1 tablespoon) chopped peanuts
2 teaspoons shredded sweetened coconut

seasonings:
⅛ teaspoon cinnamon

You'll need:
large plate

Prep: 5 minutes

1. Core apple(s), and cut into half-moon slices about ¼-inch thick. Lay slices on a large plate, and sprinkle with cinnamon.

2. Drizzle caramel over the apple slices, and top with peanuts and coconut.

MAKES 2 SERVINGS

HG TIP

If needed, microwave caramel in a small microwave-safe bowl for 15 seconds, or until soft enough to drizzle.

BLUEBERRY BLINTZADILLA

 V **Entire recipe:** 273 calories, 12g total fat (7g sat fat), 557mg sodium, 36g carbs, 7.5g fiber, 8.5g sugars, 12g protein

273 CALORIES

3 tablespoons **light/reduced-fat cream cheese**
2 tablespoons **light/low-fat ricotta cheese**
1 packet **natural no-calorie sweetener**
¼ teaspoon **vanilla extract**
1 **large high-fiber flour tortilla** with 110 calories or less
¼ cup **freeze-dried blueberries**

seasonings:
Dash cinnamon

You'll need: medium bowl, skillet, nonstick spray

Prep: 5 minutes
Cook: 5 minutes

1. In a medium bowl, add cream cheese, ricotta cheese, sweetener, vanilla extract, and cinnamon. Mix until uniform.

2. Spread onto the tortilla, and top with blueberries.

3. Fold the tortilla in half, and gently press to seal.

4. Bring a skillet sprayed with nonstick spray to medium-high heat. Cook until hot and crispy, about 2 minutes per side.

5. Slice into wedges.

MAKES 1 SERVING

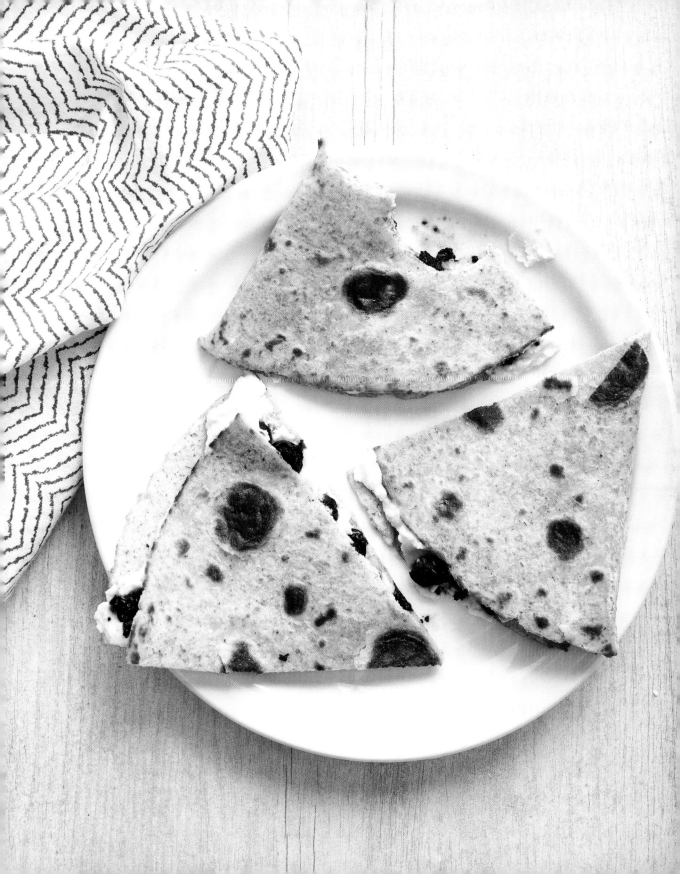

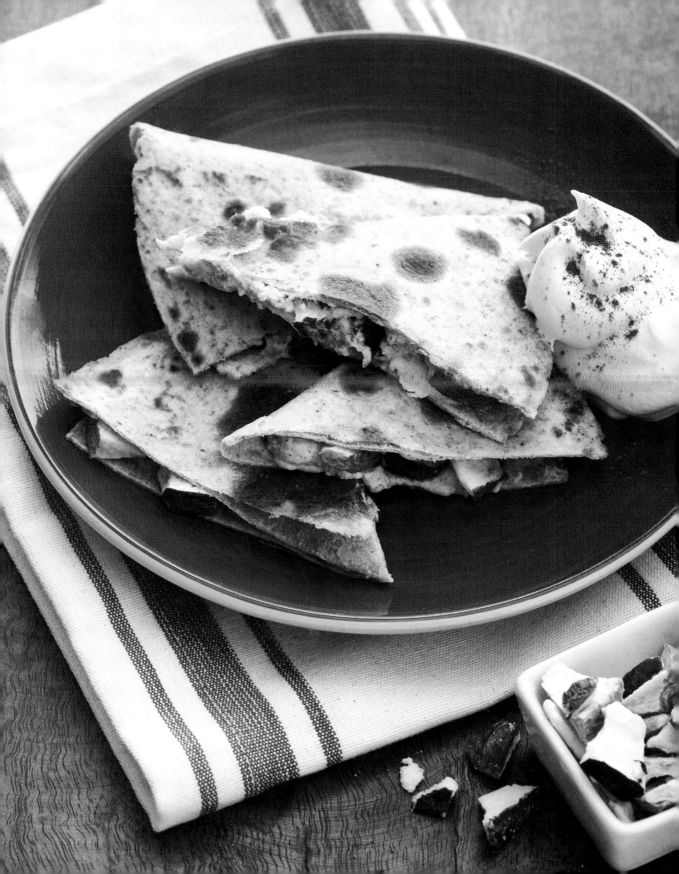

APPLE CINNAMON BLINTZADILLA

 Entire recipe: 282 calories, 12g total fat (7g sat fat), 570mg sodium, 38g carbs, 7.5g fiber, 11g sugars, 11.5g protein

6

3 tablespoons **light/reduced-fat cream cheese**
2 tablespoons **light/low-fat ricotta cheese**
1 packet **natural no-calorie sweetener**
¼ teaspoon **vanilla extract**
1 **large high-fiber flour tortilla** with 110 calories or less
⅓ cup chopped **freeze-dried apples**

seasonings:
⅛ teaspoon cinnamon

You'll need: medium bowl, skillet, nonstick spray

Prep: 5 minutes
Cook: 5 minutes

1. In a medium bowl, combine cream cheese, ricotta cheese, sweetener, vanilla extract, and cinnamon. Mix until uniform.

2. Spread onto the tortilla, and top with apples.

3. Fold the tortilla in half, and gently press to seal.

4. Bring a skillet sprayed with nonstick spray to medium-high heat. Cook until hot and crispy, about 2 minutes per side.

5. Slice into wedges.

MAKES 1 SERVING

PINEAPPLE CHEESECAKE DIP

 ⅙th of recipe (about ¼ cup): 82 calories, 3g total fat (2.5g sat fat), 82mg sodium, 11g carbs, 0.5g fiber, 8.5g sugars, 2g protein

6

¼ cup **light/reduced-fat cream cheese**
One 8-ounce can **crushed pineapple packed in juice,**
   thoroughly drained
¾ cup **natural light whipped topping**
⅓ cup **fat-free plain Greek yogurt**
1 packet **natural no-calorie sweetener**
1 teaspoon **vanilla extract**

seasonings:
¼ teaspoon cinnamon
Dash salt

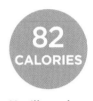

You'll need:
medium bowl

Prep: 5 minutes

In a medium bowl, stir cream cheese until smooth. Add all ingredients and seasonings. Mix until uniform.

MAKES 6 SERVINGS

6 SIMPLE CHEESECAKE DIPPERS

1. **Pretzels**

2. **Apple Slices**

3. **Sugar Cones (break 'em up or fill 'em up!)**

4. **Graham Crackers**

5. **Strawberries**

6. **Your Spoon!**

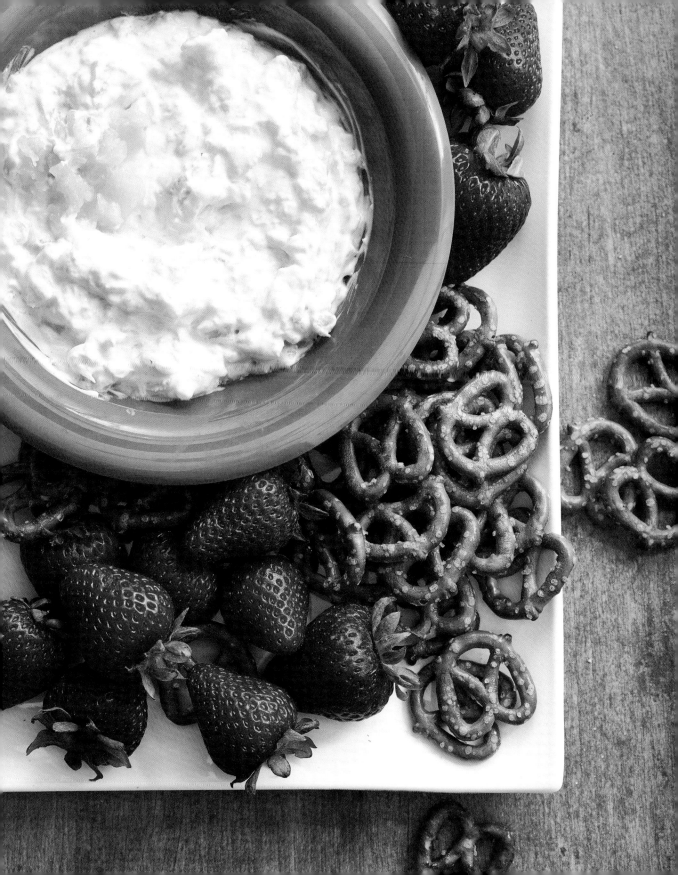

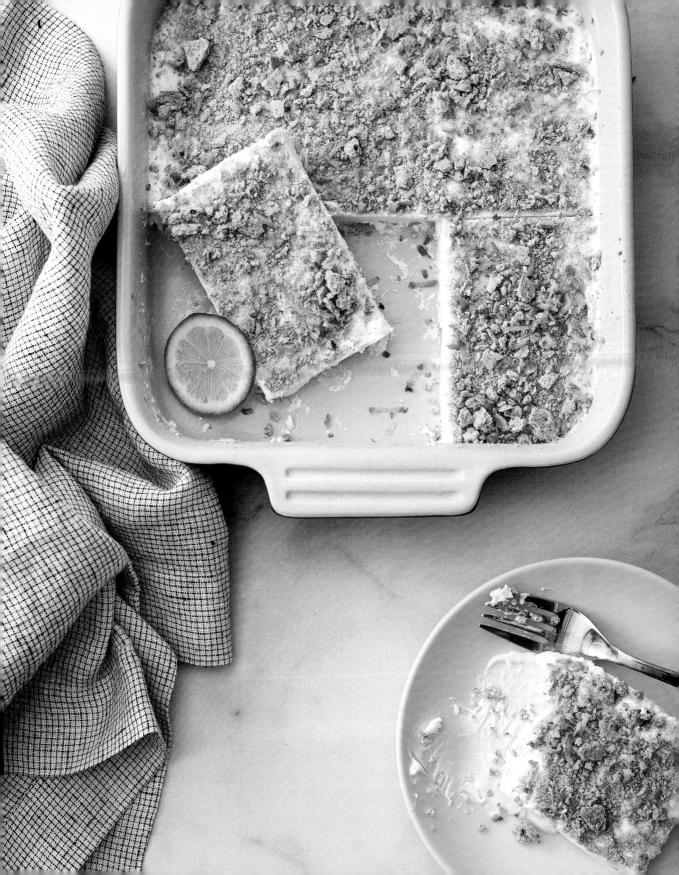

FREEZY LIME BARS

⅙th of pan: 134 calories, 6g total fat (4g sat fat), 142mg sodium, 18g carbs, 0.5g fiber, 8g sugars, 7.5g protein

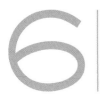

½ cup **light/reduced-fat cream cheese**
2 **limes**
1½ cups **fat-free plain Greek yogurt**
1 cup **natural light whipped topping**
2 tablespoons **Truvia spoonable no-calorie sweetener**
2 sheets (8 crackers) **graham crackers**, finely crushed

134 CALORIES

You'll need: large bowl, fine grater or zester, 8-inch by 8-inch baking pan

Prep: 10 minutes
Freeze: 3½ hours

1. Place cream cheese in a large bowl, and stir until smooth.

2. Add 1 teaspoon lime zest and 3 tablespoons lime juice.

3. Add all remaining ingredients *except* graham crackers. Mix until smooth and uniform.

4. Transfer to an 8-inch by 8-inch baking pan, and smooth out the top. Sprinkle with crushed graham crackers.

5. Cover and freeze until firm, at least 3½ hours.

6. Top with any leftover lime zest.

MAKES 6 SERVINGS

CHEESECAKE STUFFED STRAWBERRIES

NC **15m** **V** **GF** **½ of recipe (5 stuffed strawberries):** 123 calories, 6g total fat (4.5g sat fat), 71mg sodium, 17g carbs, 2g fiber, 11g sugars, 2g protein

2 tablespoons **light/reduced-fat cream cheese**
⅓ cup **natural light whipped topping**
1 packet **natural no-calorie sweetener**
¼ teaspoon **vanilla extract**
2 teaspoons **mini semi-sweet chocolate chips**
10 large **strawberries**

123 CALORIES

You'll need: medium bowl, narrow spoon, plastic bag

Prep: 10 minutes

1. To make the filling, in a medium bowl, stir cream cheese until smooth. Add all remaining ingredients *except* chocolate chips and strawberries. Mix until smooth and uniform. Fold in 1 teaspoon chocolate chips.

2. Slice the stem ends off the strawberries, about ½ inch below the stem, revealing an opening in each berry. Use a narrow spoon to remove about half of the flesh inside each berry, allowing room for filling.

3. Spoon filling into the bottom corner of a plastic bag, snip off the tip of that corner to create a small hole, and pipe mixture through the hole into the strawberries. Top with remaining 1 teaspoon chocolate chips.

MAKES 2 SERVINGS

HG TIPS

- **Cut a thin slice off the bottom of each strawberry, so the berries sit flat.**
- **Use a grapefruit spoon to scoop out the flesh!**

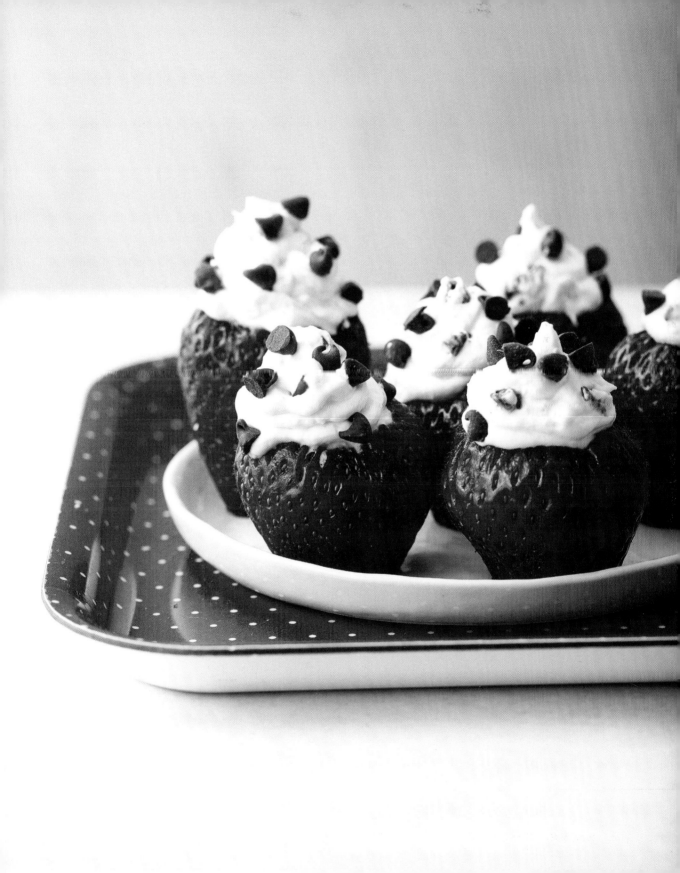

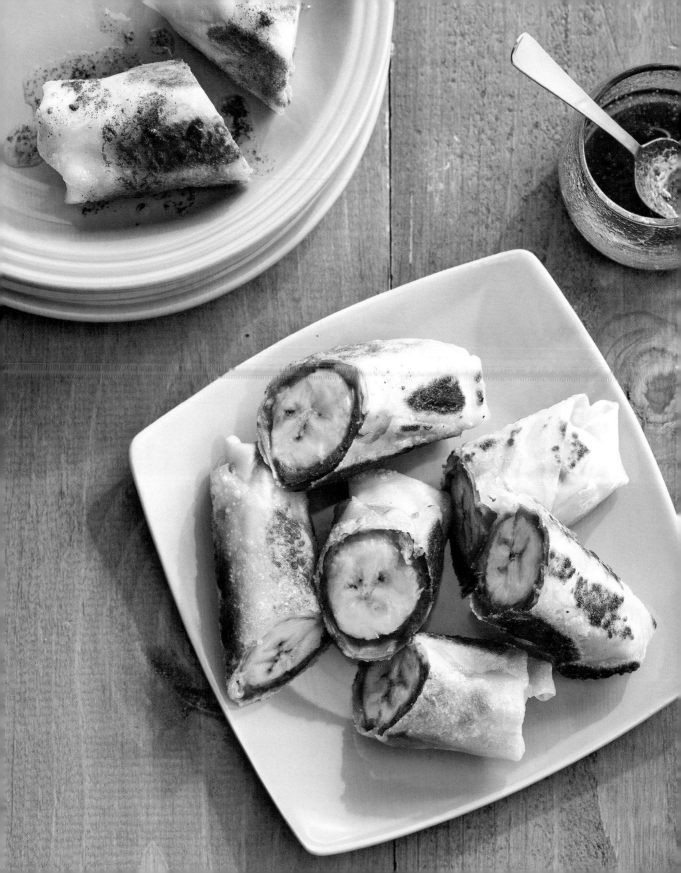

BANANARAMA EGG ROLLS

 V **¼th of recipe (1 egg roll):** 166 calories, 4.5g total fat (1.5g sat fat), 143mg sodium, 29.5g carbs, 2.5g fiber, 9.5g sugars, 4.5g protein

6

2 **medium bananas**
1½ tablespoons **powdered peanut butter**
2 teaspoons **creamy peanut butter**
1 teaspoon **honey**
4 **square egg roll wrappers**
1½ tablespoons **whipped butter**

seasonings:
¼ teaspoon cinnamon

166 CALORIES

You'll need:
2 small bowls (one microwave-safe), skillet, nonstick spray

Prep: 5 minutes
Cook: 10 minutes

1. Slice bananas in half widthwise, for a total of 4 pieces.

2. In a small bowl, combine both types of peanut butter with 1½ tablespoons water. Add honey, and mix until smooth and uniform.

3. Lay an egg roll wrapper flat on a dry surface. Place a banana half a little below the center of the wrapper. Spread ¼th of the peanut butter mixture over top and sides of the banana.

4. Moisten all four edges by dabbing your fingers in water and going over the edges smoothly. Fold the sides about ¾ inch toward the middle to keep banana in place. Roll up the wrapper around the banana, and continue to the top. Seal with a dab of water.

5. Repeat to make three more egg rolls.

6. In a small microwave-safe bowl, mix butter with cinnamon. Microwave for 10 seconds, or until melted. Evenly brush over egg rolls.

7. Bring a skillet sprayed with nonstick spray to medium heat. Rotating occasionally, cook egg rolls until golden brown and crispy, about 6 minutes.

MAKES 4 SERVINGS

HG TIPS

- **Find egg roll wrappers with the tofu in the refrigerated section of the market. They're just a larger version of wonton wrappers.**

- **To freeze leftover wrappers, separate them with sheets of wax paper. Then thaw before using!**

NO-MELT BANANA SPLIT

 Entire recipe: 194 calories, 5.5g fat (2.5g sat fat), 6mg sodium, 37g carbs, 4.5g fiber, 22g sugars, 3g protein

5

1 **medium banana**
2 teaspoons **mini semi-sweet chocolate chips**
1 teaspoon **unsweetened vanilla almond milk**
2 tablespoons chopped **freeze-dried strawberries**
2 teaspoons chopped **peanuts**

194 CALORIES

You'll need:
large plate, small microwave-safe bowl

Prep: 5 minutes
Cook: 5 minutes or less

1. Slice banana into coins, about ½-inch thick. Place on a large plate.

2. In a small microwave-safe bowl, combine chocolate chips with milk.

3. Microwave at 50 percent power for 25 seconds.

4. Stir until smooth and uniform. Drizzle over banana.

5. Sprinkle with strawberries and peanuts.

MAKES 1 SERVING

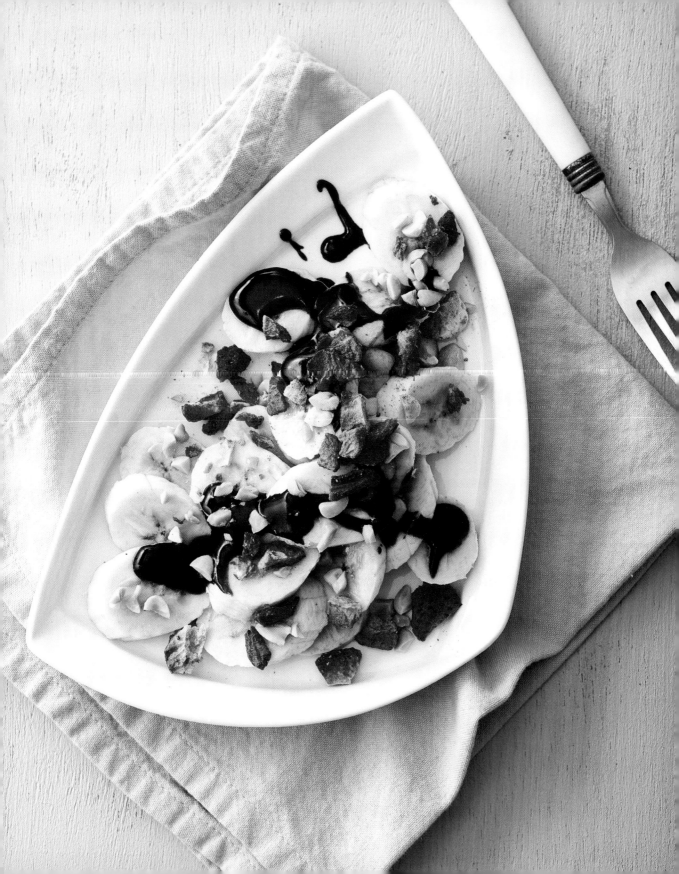

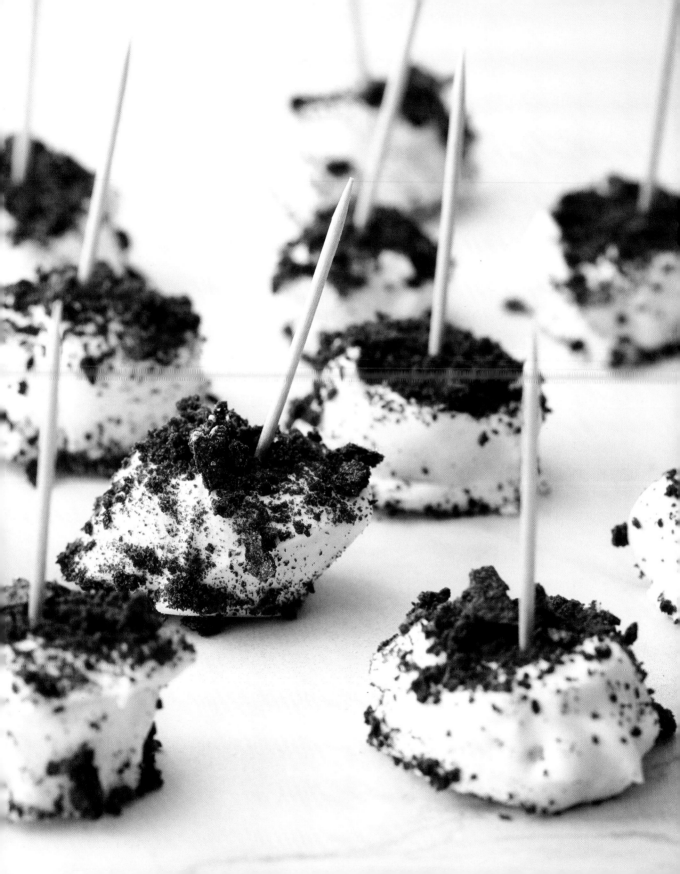

COOKIES & CREAM BANANA BITES

 ¼th of recipe (6 pieces): 105 calories, 2g total fat (1.5g sat fat), 33mg sodium, 22g carbs, 1.5g fiber, 12g sugars, 1.5g protein

4

½ cup **natural light whipped topping**
¼ cup **fat-free vanilla yogurt**
2 **medium bananas**, sliced into 24 coins
1 sheet (4 crackers) **chocolate graham crackers**, crushed

105 CALORIES

You'll need: baking sheet (or large plate), parchment paper, medium bowl, toothpicks

Prep: 15 minutes
Freeze: 1 hour
15 minutes

1. Line a baking sheet (or large plate) with parchment paper.

2. In a medium bowl, mix whipped topping with yogurt.

3. Dip banana coins in yogurt mixture. Using a spoon (or your fingers), rotate to generously coat.

4. Transfer to the baking sheet. Repeat with remaining banana coins, evenly spacing them out on the sheet.

5. Sprinkle with crushed graham crackers.

6. Insert toothpicks into the centers of each coin.

7. Freeze until yogurt is firm, about 1 hour.

MAKES 4 SERVINGS

NUTTY 'N NICE CREAM CONES

 ¼th of recipe: 174 calories, 6g total fat (3.5g sat fat), 90mg sodium, 27.5g carbs, 2g fiber, 13g sugars, 5g protein

6
- ½ cup (about 1 medium) mashed **extra-ripe banana**
- ¼ cup **powdered peanut butter**
- 2 tablespoons **light/reduced-fat cream cheese**
- 1 cup **natural light whipped topping**
- 4 **sugar cones**
- 2 teaspoons chopped **peanuts**

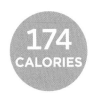
174 CALORIES

You'll need:
medium-large bowl

Prep: 10 minutes

1. In a medium-large bowl, combine banana, powdered peanut butter, and cream cheese. Mix until uniform.

2. Fold in whipped topping.

3. Spoon mixture into the cones. (See HG Tip.)

4. Top with peanuts.

MAKES 4 SERVINGS

HG TIP

For beautiful swirls, use a piping bag! Need a DIY version? Transfer the filling to a plastic bag, and squeeze it down toward a bottom corner. Snip off the corner with scissors, creating a small hole for piping.

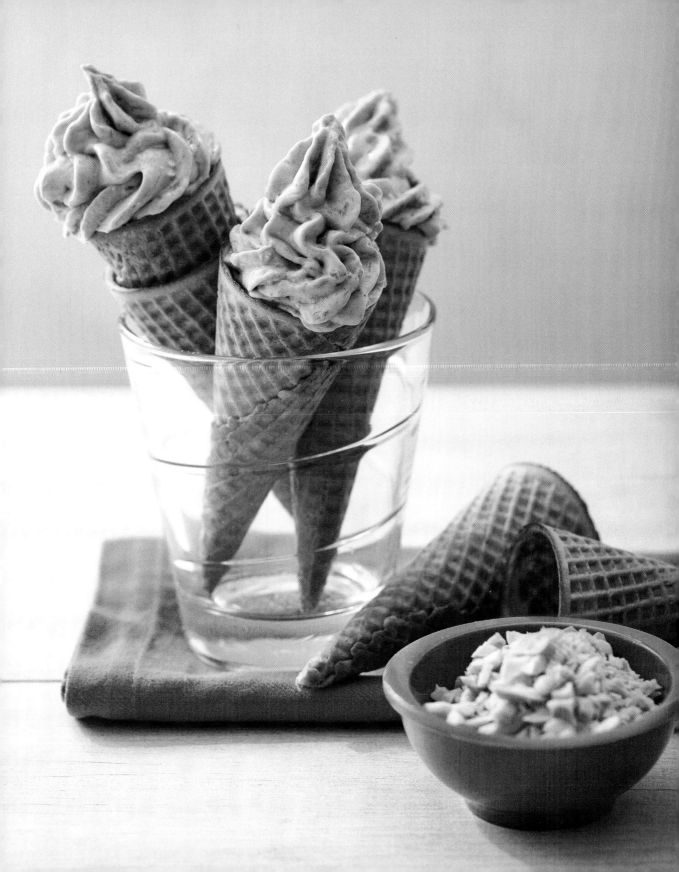

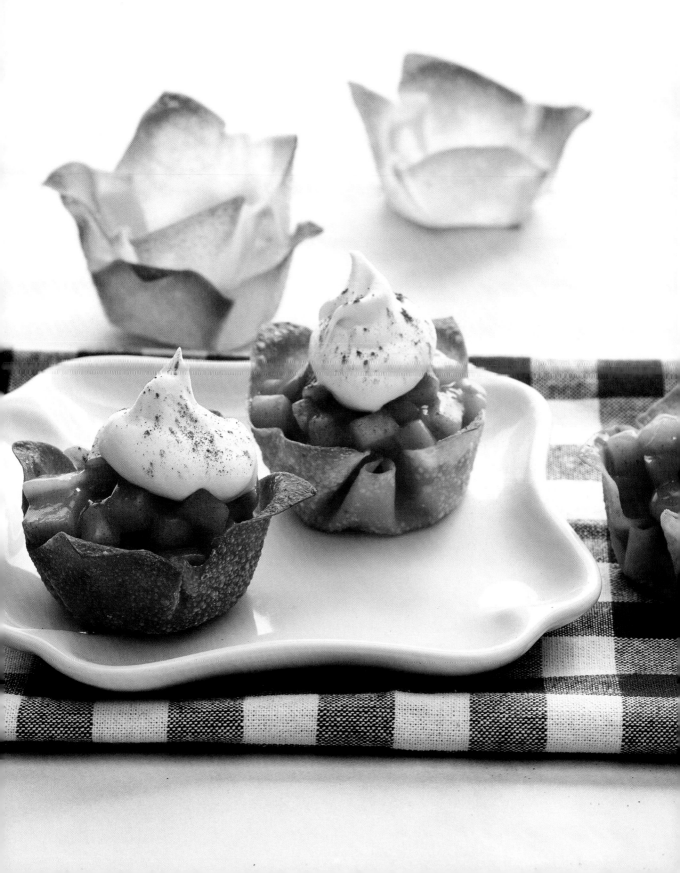

PERSONAL PEACH PIES

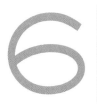

¹⁄₁₂th of recipe (1 mini pie): 47 calories, 0.5g total fat (<0.5g sat fat), 55mg sodium, 10g carbs, 1g fiber, 4.5g sugars, 1g protein

6

12 **square wonton wrappers**
1 tablespoon **cornstarch**
3 cups finely chopped **peaches** (fresh or thawed from frozen; no sugar added)
2 tablespoons **brown sugar** (not packed)
1 packet **natural no-calorie sweetener**
1 tablespoon **whipped butter**, room temperature

seasonings:
½ teaspoon cinnamon, or more for topping
Dash salt

47 CALORIES

You'll need: 12-cup muffin pan, nonstick spray, nonstick pot

Prep: 15 minutes
Cook: 10 minutes

1. Preheat oven to 350 degrees. Spray a 12-cup muffin pan with nonstick spray.

2. Press a wonton wrapper into each cup of the muffin pan. Lightly spray with nonstick spray. Bake until lightly browned, about 8 minutes.

3. Meanwhile, in a nonstick pot, combine cornstarch with ½ cup water, and stir to dissolve. Add peaches, brown sugar, sweetener, and seasonings. Set heat to medium. Stirring frequently, cook until peaches have slightly softened and mixture is thick and gooey, 6 to 8 minutes.

4. Remove from heat, and stir in butter. Evenly fill wonton cups, about 3 tablespoons each.

MAKES 12 SERVINGS

HG TIP

If you're not serving these right away, store the wonton cups at room temp in a sealable container or bag, and refrigerate the filling in a sealed container.

TEENY-TINY LEMON CREAM PIES

(V) **⅕th of recipe (3 mini pies):** 96 calories, 4.5g total fat (2.5g sat fat), 85mg sodium, 12g carbs, 0.5g fiber, 3.5g sugars, 3g protein

1 lemon
¼ cup light/reduced-fat cream cheese
½ cup natural light whipped topping
¼ cup fat-free vanilla Greek yogurt
1 packet natural no-calorie sweetener
15 frozen mini fillo shells

96 CALORIES

You'll need: fine grater or zester, medium bowl, baking sheet

Prep: 10 minutes
Cook: 5 minutes
Chill: 1 hour

1. Add 1 teaspoon lemon zest and 1 tablespoon lemon juice into a medium bowl.

2. Add cream cheese and stir until smooth. Add all remaining ingredients except fillo shells. Stir until smooth and uniform. Cover and refrigerate for 1 hour, or until chilled.

3. Preheat oven to 350 degrees.

4. Bake shells on a baking sheet until lightly browned and crispy, about 5 minutes.

5. Just before serving, evenly distribute filling into the fillo shells.

6. Top with any leftover lemon zest.

MAKES 5 SERVINGS

HG TIP

Not serving these right away? Store the baked fillo shells at room temp in a sealable container or bag, and refrigerate the filling in a sealed container.

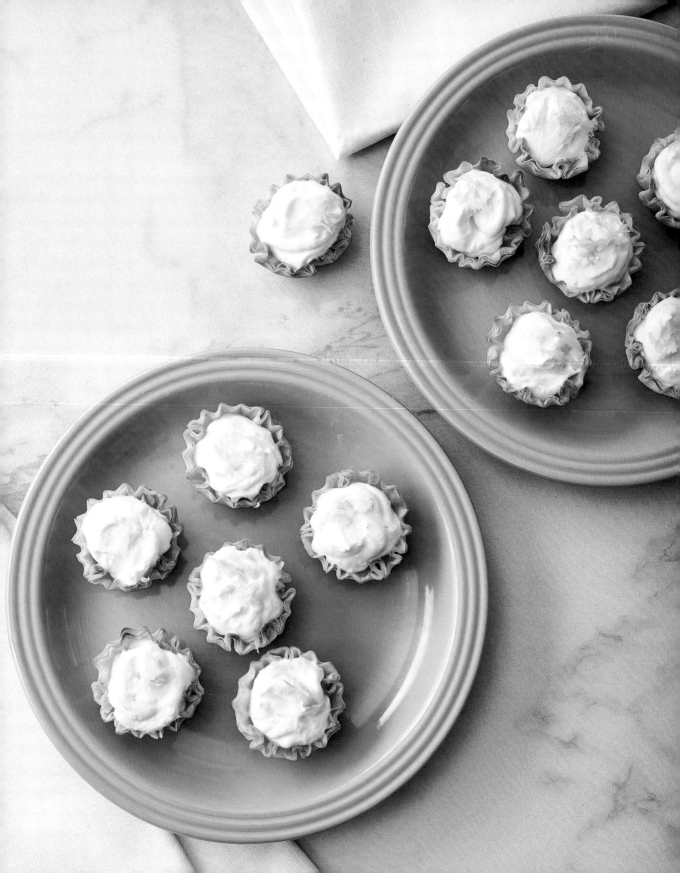

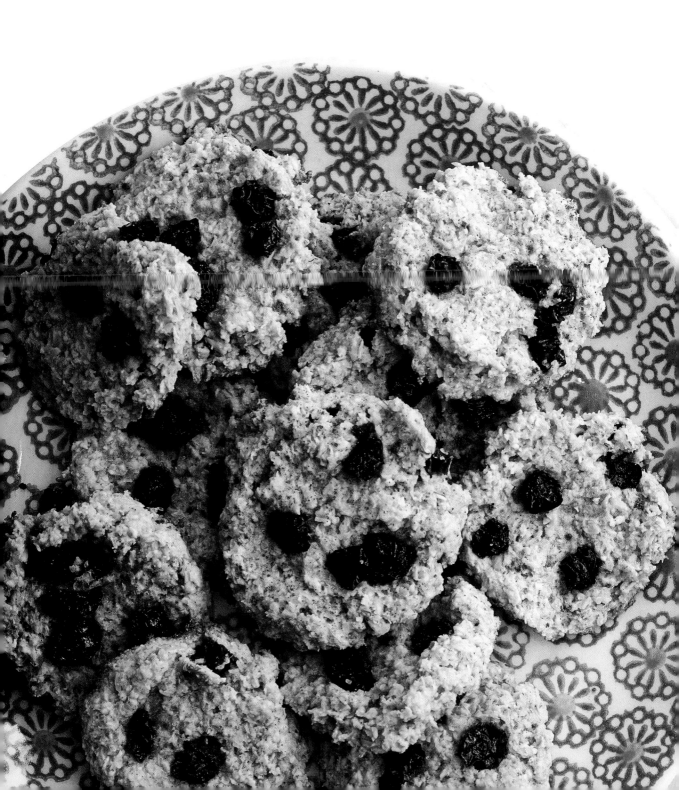

9

SIMPLY MORE . . . SWEETS!

Face it: If dessert isn't easy, you just might reach for the first thing you see, which could be a bad choice! That's where these super sweets with short ingredient lists come in! Chocolate, cheesecake, peanut butter, and beyond . . .

SIMPLE WONTON CRUNCHERS

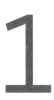 **1/12th of recipe (1 cruncher):** 19 calories, 0g total fat (0g sat fat), 35mg sodium, 4g carbs, <0.5g fiber, <0.5g sugars, 0.5g protein

1

| 12 **square wonton wrappers**

19 CALORIES

You'll need: 12-cup muffin pan, nonstick spray

Prep: 5 minutes
Cook: 10 minutes

1. Preheat oven to 350 degrees. Spray a 12-cup muffin pan with nonstick spray.

2. Press a wonton wrapper into each cup of the muffin pan. Lightly spray with nonstick spray. Bake until lightly browned, about 8 minutes.

MAKES 12 SERVINGS

HG FYI

You can even use these for SAVORY snacks, like my Tiny Taco Salads! Recipe at Hungry-Girl.com . . .

Mix 'n Match Fillings

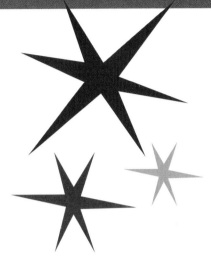

Creamy

- Fat-free yogurt (regular or Greek)
- Light whipped topping
- Light ice cream

Crunchy

- Crushed graham crackers
- Sliced or chopped nuts
- Crushed pretzels

Fruity

- Fresh fruit (berries, cherries & more)
- Freeze-dried fruit
- Fruit preserves (mix with water for a yummy sauce)

Fun

- Sprinkles
- Shredded coconut
- Mini chocolate chips

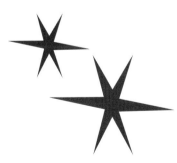

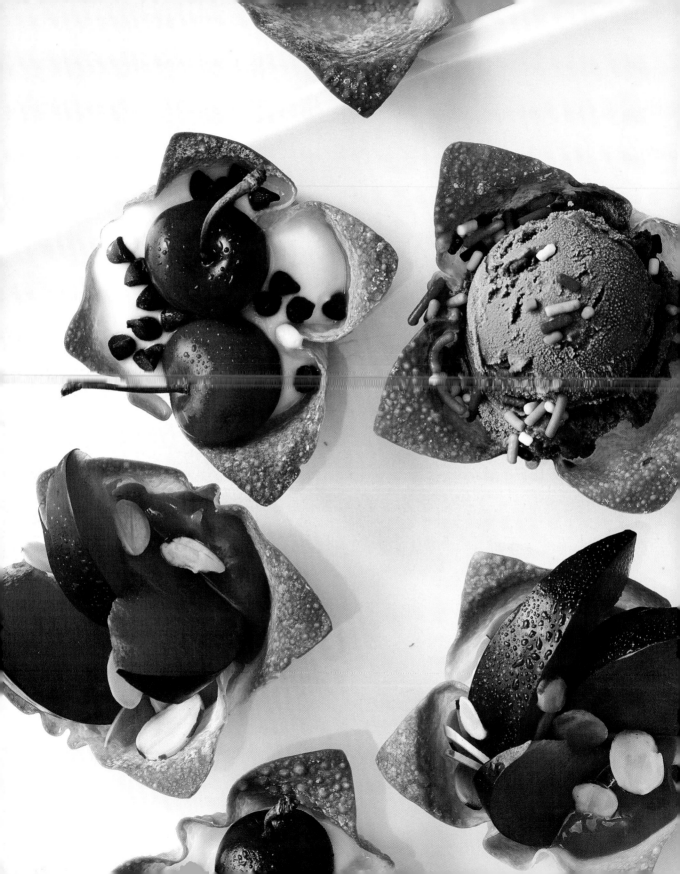

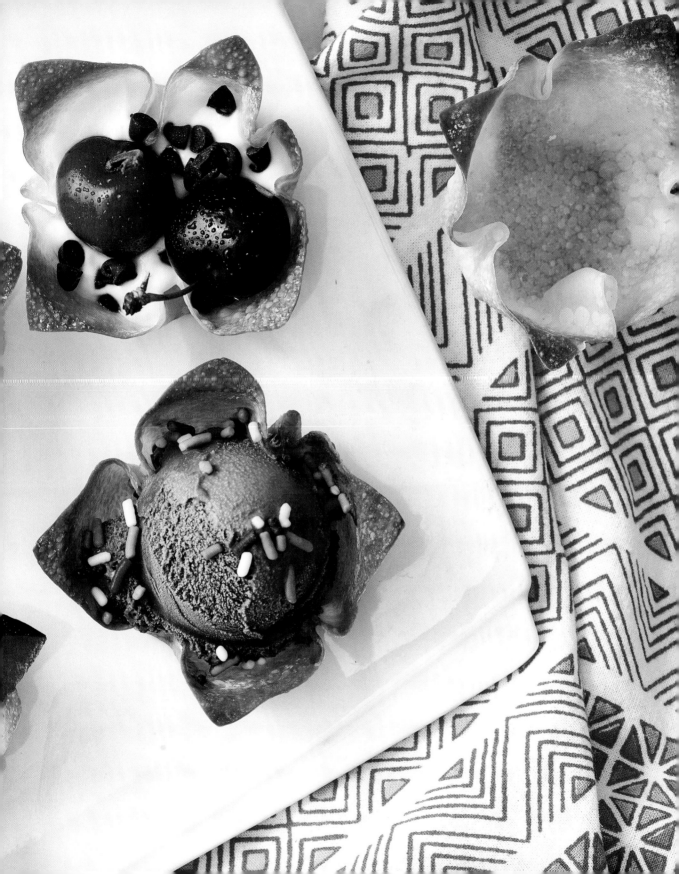

CANNOLI CRUNCHERS

 ¹⁄₁₂th of recipe (1 cruncher): 120 calories, 5g total fat (4g sat fat), 100mg sodium, 15g carbs, 0.5g fiber, 8.5g sugars, 5g protein

6

12 **square wonton wrappers**
2¼ cups **light/low-fat ricotta cheese**
2 cups **natural light whipped topping**
4 packets **natural no-calorie sweetener**
½ teaspoon **vanilla extract**
¼ cup **mini semi-sweet chocolate chips**

You'll need: 12-cup muffin pan, nonstick spray, large bowl

Prep: 10 minutes
Cook: 10 minutes
Cool: 10 minutes

1. Preheat oven to 350 degrees. Spray a 12-cup muffin pan with nonstick spray.

2. Press a wonton wrapper into each cup of the muffin pan. Lightly spray with nonstick spray. Bake until lightly browned, about 10 minutes.

3. Let cool completely, about 10 minutes.

4. Meanwhile, in a large bowl, thoroughly mix ricotta, whipped topping, sweetener, and vanilla extract.

5. Stir in 2 tablespoons chocolate chips. Evenly distribute mixture among the wonton cups.

6. Top with remaining 2 tablespoons chocolate chips.

MAKES 12 SERVINGS

HG TIP

Nobody likes soggy cannoli! Until you're ready to serve, store the baked wonton cups at room temp in a sealable container or bag, and refrigerate the filling in a sealed container.

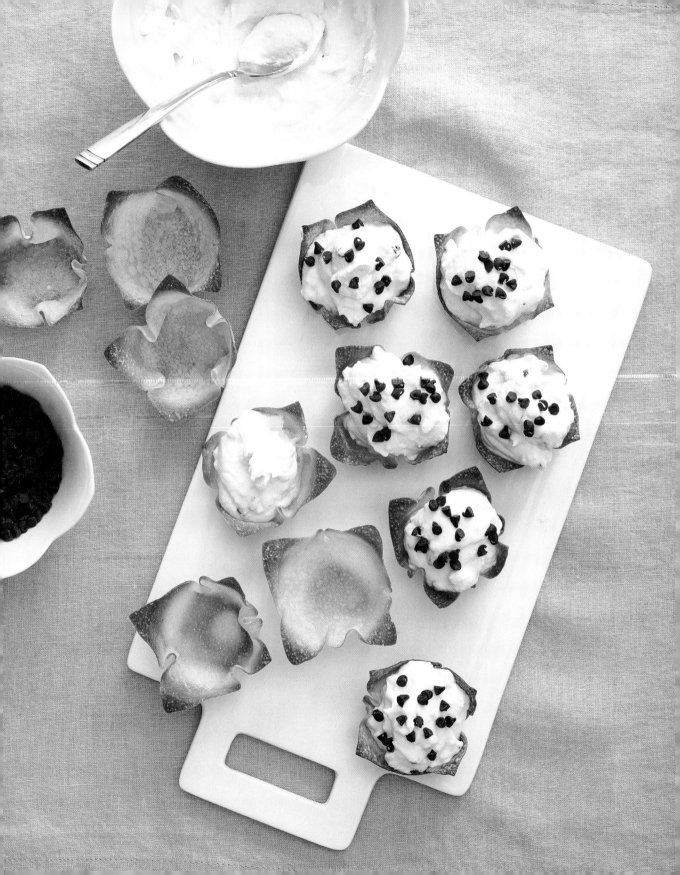

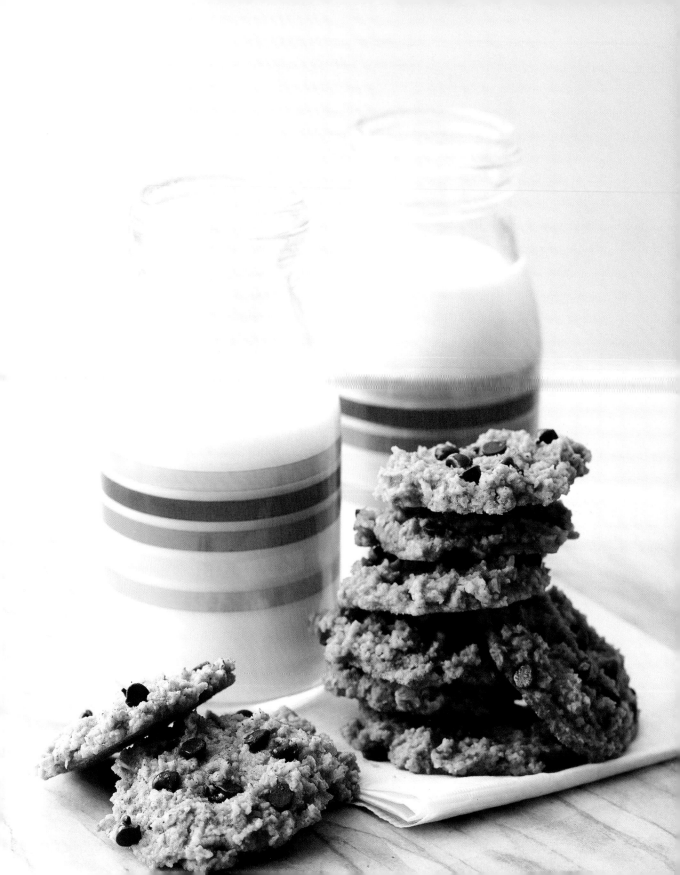

CHOCOLATE CHIP COOKIES

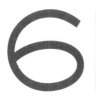 **30m** **V** **GF** **¹⁄₁₂th of recipe (1 cookie):** 47 calories, 2g total fat (1g sat fat), 33mg sodium, 6.5g carbs, 1g fiber, 1.5g sugars, 1g protein

6

1 cup **old-fashioned oats**
½ cup **unsweetened applesauce**
2 tablespoons **whipped butter**, room temperature
2 packets **natural no-calorie sweetener**
1 teaspoon **vanilla extract**
1 tablespoon **mini semi-sweet chocolate chips**

seasonings:
¼ teaspoon cinnamon
⅛ teaspoon salt

47 CALORIES

You'll need: baking sheet, nonstick spray, small blender or food processor, medium-large bowl

Prep: 10 minutes
Cook: 20 minutes

1. Preheat oven to 350 degrees. Spray a baking sheet with nonstick spray.

2. In a small blender or food processor, pulse oats to the consistency of coarse flour. Transfer to a medium-large bowl.

3. Add all remaining ingredients and seasonings *except* chocolate chips. Mix until uniform.

4. Stir in ½ tablespoon of chocolate chips.

5. Evenly distribute mixture into 12 mounds on the baking sheet, about 1½ tablespoons each. Use the back of a spoon to spread and flatten into 2-inch circles.

6. Top with remaining ½ tablespoon chocolate chips, and lightly press to adhere.

7. Bake until a knife inserted into the center of a cookie comes out clean, 16 to 18 minutes.

MAKES 12 SERVINGS

SURVEY SAYS . . .

It's almost a tie! 51% of Hungry Girl fans would rather eat cookies than cookie dough. There's no egg in this batter, so you could eat both!

PB SURPRISE COOKIES

 30m **V** **GF** **¹⁄₁₆th of recipe (1 cookie):** 51 calories, 1.5g total fat (<0.5g sat fat), 26mg sodium, 8g carbs, 1.5g fiber, 2g sugars, 2g protein

6

1 cup (about 2 medium) mashed **extra-ripe bananas**
1 cup **old-fashioned oats**
⅓ cup **powdered peanut butter**
1½ tablespoons **creamy peanut butter**
2 teaspoons **vanilla extract**
2 packets **natural no-calorie sweetener**

seasonings:
½ teaspoon cinnamon
⅛ teaspoon salt

51 CALORIES

You'll need: baking sheet, nonstick spray, medium-large bowl

Prep: 10 minutes
Cook: 15 minutes

1. Preheat oven to 350 degrees. Spray a baking sheet with nonstick spray.

2. In a medium-large bowl, combine all ingredients and seasonings. Add ⅓ cup water, and mix until uniform.

3. Evenly distribute mixture into 16 mounds on the baking sheet, about 1½ tablespoons each. Use the back of a spoon to spread and flatten into 2-inch circles.

4. Bake until a knife inserted into the center of a cookie comes out clean, about 14 minutes.

MAKES 16 SERVINGS

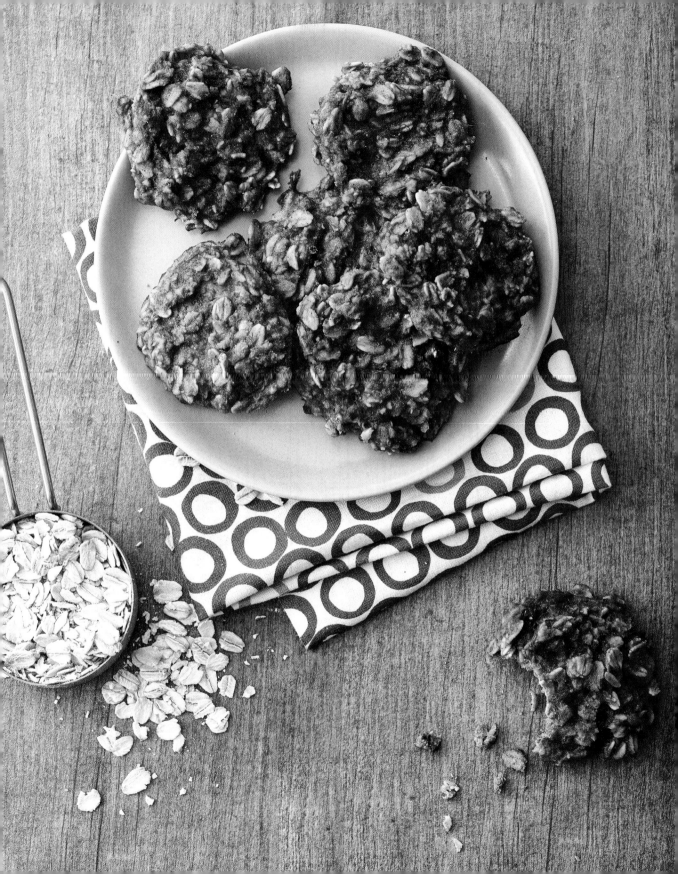

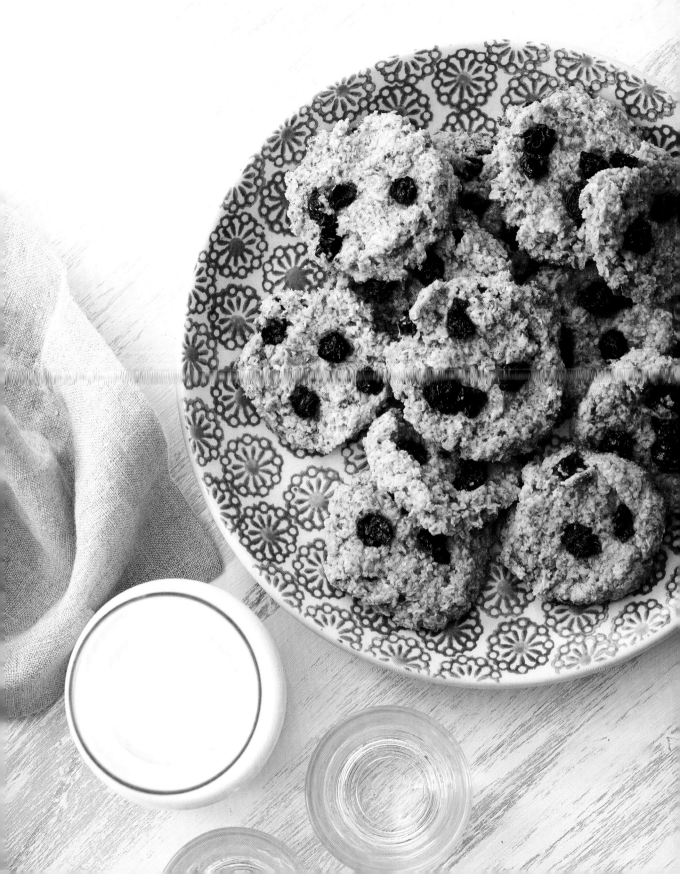

OATMEAL RAISIN COOKIES

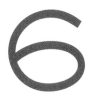

¹⁄₁₂th of recipe (1 cookie): 49 calories, 1.5g total fat (0.5g sat fat), 33mg sodium, 7g carbs, 1g fiber, 2g sugars, 1g protein

6

2 tablespoons **raisins**, chopped
1 cup **old-fashioned oats**
½ cup **unsweetened applesauce**
2 tablespoons **whipped butter**, room temperature
2 packets **natural no-calorie sweetener**
1 teaspoon **vanilla extract**

seasonings:
½ teaspoon pumpkin pie spice
⅛ teaspoon salt

49 CALORIES

You'll need: baking sheet, nonstick spray, small bowl, blender or food processor, medium-large bowl

Prep: 15 minutes
Cook: 20 minutes

1. Preheat oven to 350 degrees. Spray a baking sheet with nonstick spray.

2. Place chopped raisins in a small bowl, and cover with warm water. Soak until softened, 5 to 10 minutes. Drain excess liquid.

3. Meanwhile, in a blender or food processor, pulse oats to the consistency of coarse flour. Transfer to a medium-large bowl.

4. Add all remaining ingredients and seasonings *except* raisins. Mix until uniform.

5. Stir in half of the raisins.

6. Evenly distribute mixture into 12 mounds on the baking sheet, about 1½ tablespoons each. Use the back of a spoon to spread and flatten into 2-inch circles.

7. Top with remaining raisins, and lightly press to adhere.

8. Bake until a knife inserted into the center of a cookie comes out clean, 16 to 18 minutes.

MAKES 12 SERVINGS

PB MIDNIGHT FUDGE BITES

 ½₀th of recipe (1 piece): 67 calories, 4g total fat (0.5g sat fat), 55mg sodium, 11g carbs, 3g fiber, 1g sugars, 3.5g protein

5

2 cups **canned pure pumpkin**
1 cup **unsweetened dark cocoa powder**, or more for topping
½ cup **creamy peanut butter**
½ cup **powdered peanut butter**
½ cup **Truvia spoonable no-calorie sweetener**

You'll need: 8-inch by 8-inch baking pan, parchment paper, food processor

Prep: 5 minutes
Cook: 30 minutes
Cool: 1 hour
Chill: 2 hours

1. Preheat oven to 350 degrees. Line an 8-inch by 8-inch baking pan with parchment paper.

2. Place all ingredients in a food processor. Puree until completely smooth and uniform.

3. Spread mixture into the baking pan, and smooth out the top.

4. Bake until top is firm, 25 to 27 minutes.

5. Let cool completely, about 1 hour.

6. Cover and refrigerate until completely chilled, at least 2 hours. (This fudge is even good slightly frozen!)

MAKES 20 SERVINGS

SURVEY SAYS . . .

53% of Hungry Girl fans say peanut butter & chocolate is a better combo than PB&J. Good thing this chapter serves up BOTH!

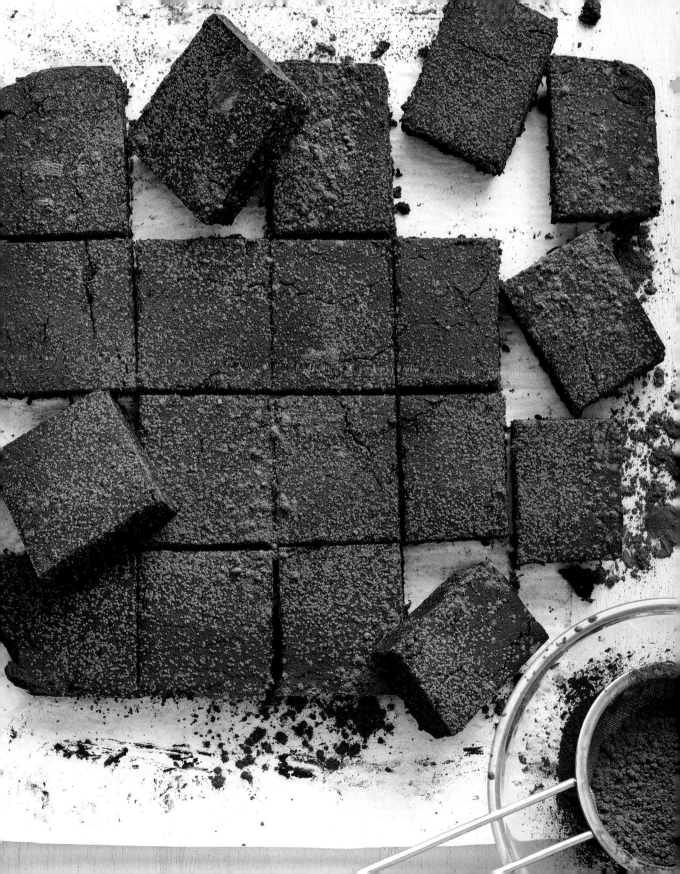

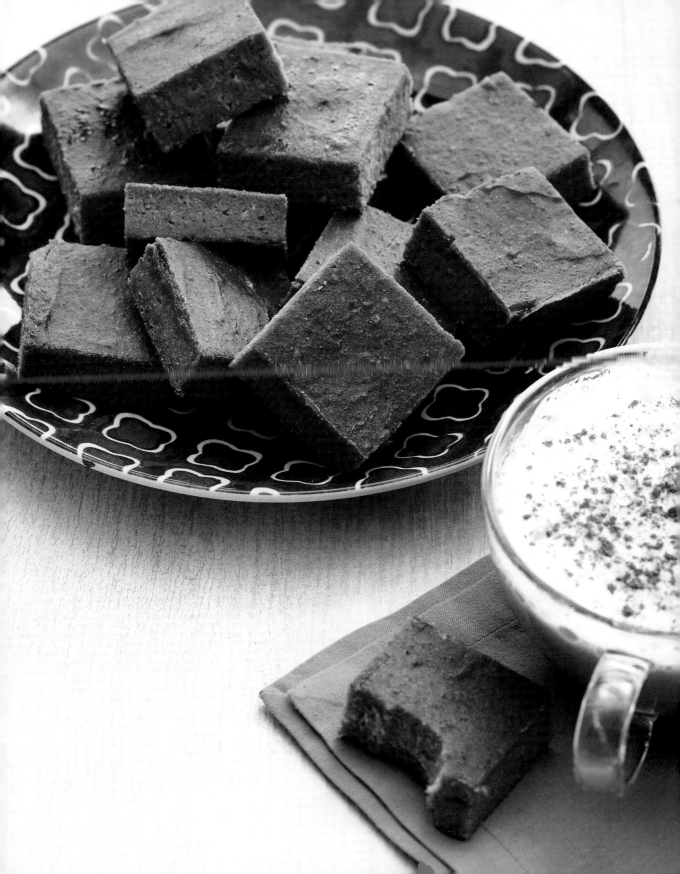

PB 'NANA FUDGE BITES

 ½₀th of recipe (1 piece): 93 calories, 5g total fat (0.5g sat fat), 28mg sodium, 10.5g carbs, 2g fiber, 3.5g sugars, 4.5g protein

4

2 cups (about 4 medium) mashed **extra-ripe bananas**
1 cup **powdered peanut butter**
⅔ cup **creamy peanut butter**
3 tablespoons **Truvia spoonable no-calorie sweetener**

93 CALORIES

You'll need: 8-inch by 8-inch baking pan, parchment paper, food processor

Prep: 10 minutes
Cook: 30 minutes
Cool: 1 hour
Chill: 2 hours

1. Preheat oven to 350 degrees. Line an 8-inch by 8-inch baking pan with parchment paper.

2. Place all ingredients in a food processor. Puree until completely smooth and uniform.

3. Transfer to the baking pan, and smooth out the top.

4. Bake until a knife inserted into the center comes out mostly clean, 25 to 30 minutes.

5. Let cool completely, about 1 hour.

6. Cover and refrigerate until completely chilled, at least 2 hours. (This fudge is even good slightly frozen!)

MAKES 20 SERVINGS

FREEZY CRUSTLESS CHEESECAKE

⅛th of recipe: 182 calories, 10g total fat (8g sat fat), 153mg sodium, 20g carbs, 0.5g fiber, 13.5g sugars, 4g protein

6

¾ cup **light/reduced-fat cream cheese**
3 cups **natural light whipped topping**
¾ cup **fat-free plain Greek yogurt**
5 packets **natural no-calorie sweetener**
1½ tablespoons **vanilla extract**
¼ cup **mini semi-sweet chocolate chips**

seasonings:
⅛ teaspoon salt

182 CALORIES

You'll need: medium bowl, 9-inch pie pan

Prep: 10 minutes
Freeze: 3 hours

1. In a medium bowl, stir cream cheese until smooth. Add all remaining ingredients and seasoning except chocolate chips. Mix until smooth and uniform.

2. Stir in 3 tablespoons chocolate chips. Transfer to a 9-inch pie pan, and smooth out the top. Top with remaining 1 tablespoon chocolate chips.

3. Cover and freeze until firm, at least 3 hours.

MAKES 8 SERVINGS

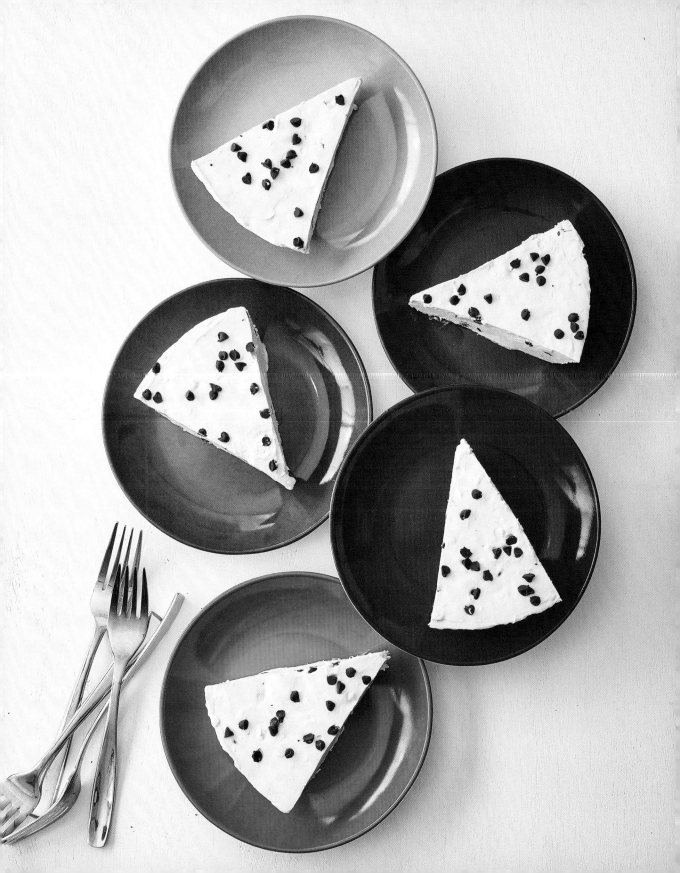

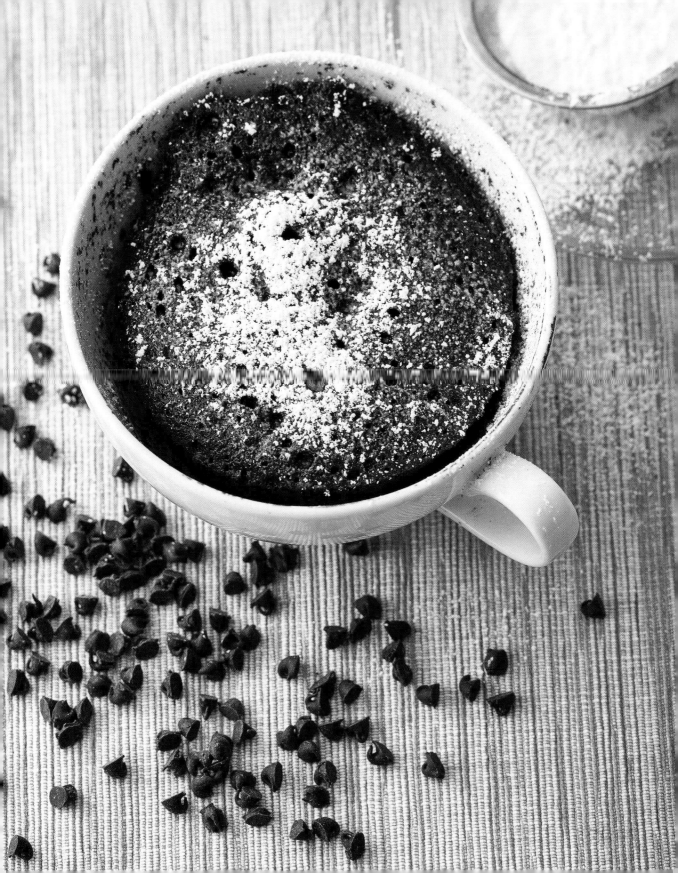

CHOCOLATE CAKE IN A MUG

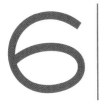 **Entire recipe:** 167 calories, 4.5g total fat (2.5g sat fat), 385mg sodium, 19g carbs, 6g fiber, 6g sugars, 12g protein

6

3 tablespoons **unsweetened cocoa powder**
3 packets **natural no-calorie sweetener**
½ teaspoon **baking powder**
⅓ cup (about 3 large) **egg whites** or **fat-free liquid egg substitute**
1 teaspoon **vanilla extract**
2 teaspoons **mini semi-sweet chocolate chips**

You'll need: large microwave-safe mug, nonstick spray

Prep: 5 minutes
Cook: 5 minutes
Cool: 10 minutes

1. Spray a large microwave safe mug with nonstick spray. Add cocoa powder, sweetener, and baking powder. Stir until uniform.

2. Add egg and vanilla extract. Whisk with a fork until just combined.

3. Stir in chocolate chips. Microwave for 2½ minutes, or until set.

4. Let cool and set for 5 to 10 minutes.

MAKES 1 SERVING

DOUBLE CHOCOLATE BROWNIES

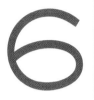

V **⅑th of recipe (1 brownie):** 115 calories, 7.5g total fat (4.5g sat fat), 174mg sodium, 20.5g carbs, 2g fiber, 2g sugars, 3g protein

½ cup **whole-wheat flour**
½ cup **unsweetened dark cocoa powder**
½ cup **Truvia spoonable no-calorie sweetener**
½ cup **whipped butter**
½ cup (about 4 large) **egg whites** or **fat-free liquid egg substitute**
2½ tablespoons **mini semi-sweet chocolate chips**

seasonings:
¼ teaspoon salt

115 CALORIES

You'll need: 8-inch by 8-inch baking pan, nonstick spray, medium-large bowl, medium microwave-safe bowl

Prep: 10 minutes
Cook: 25 minutes
Cool: 1 hour

1. Preheat oven to 350 degrees. Spray an 8-inch by 8-inch baking pan with nonstick spray.

2. In a medium-large bowl, mix flour, cocoa powder, sweetener, and salt.

3. In a medium microwave-safe bowl, microwave butter for 30 seconds, or until melted. Add egg, and whisk with a fork until uniform.

4. Add butter mixture to the medium-large bowl, and mix until uniform. (Batter will be thick.)

5. Stir in 1 tablespoon chocolate chips. Transfer to the baking pan, and smooth out the top.

6. Top with remaining 1½ tablespoons chocolate chips, and lightly press to adhere.

7. Bake until a knife inserted into the center comes out mostly clean, 20 to 25 minutes.

8. Let cool completely, about 1 hour.

MAKES 9 SERVINGS

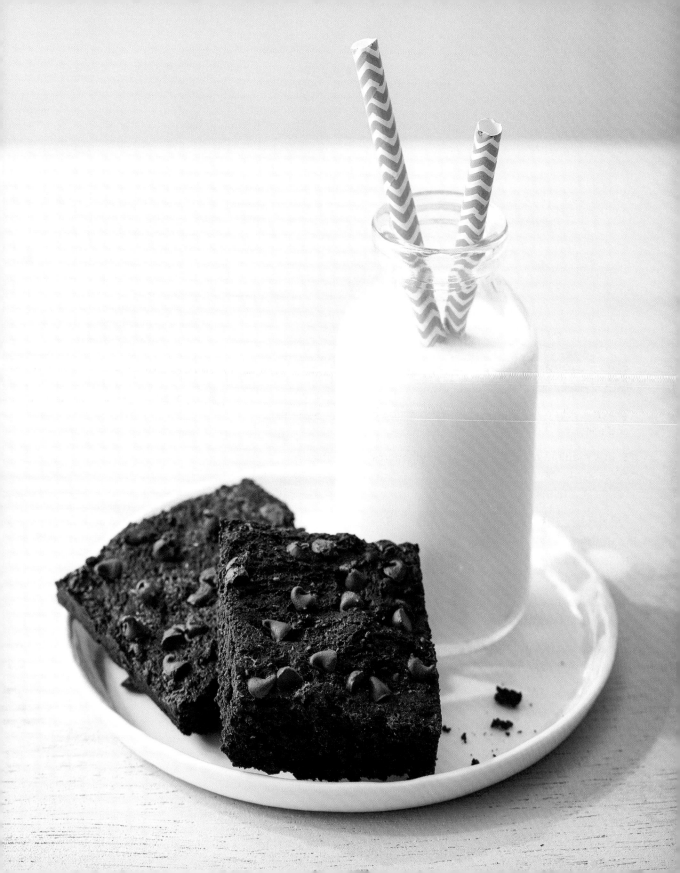

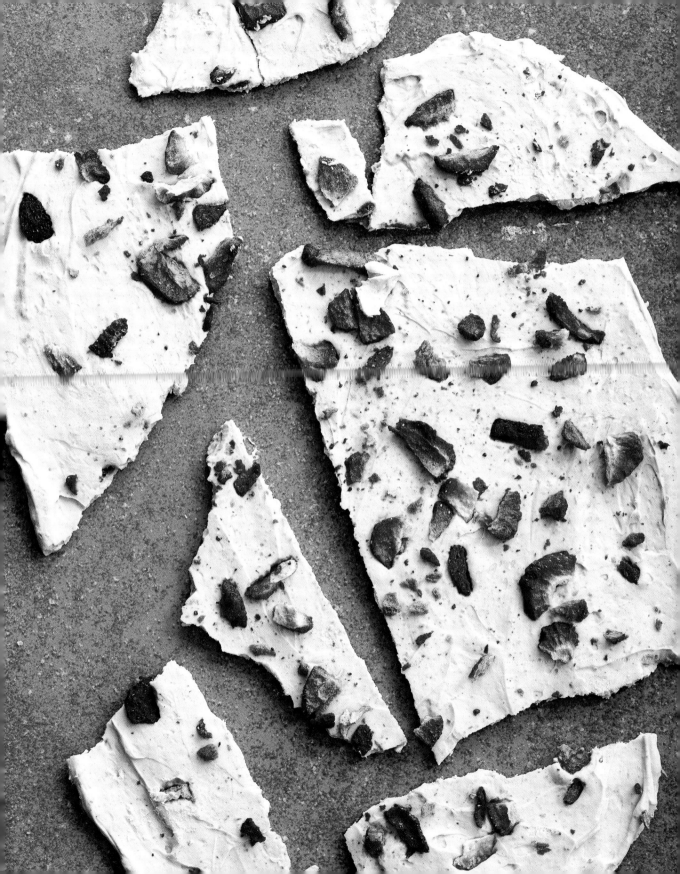

PB&J FROZEN YOGURT BARK

 ⅙th of recipe (1 piece): 87 calories, 4g total fat (1.5g sat fat), 27mg sodium, 8g carbs, 1g fiber, 4.5g sugars, 5g protein

6

¾ cup **fat-free plain Greek yogurt**
¾ cup **natural light whipped topping**
2 tablespoons **creamy peanut butter**
2 tablespoons **powdered peanut butter**
1 packet **natural no-calorie sweetener**
3 tablespoons chopped **freeze-dried strawberries**

87 CALORIES

You'll need: 8-inch by 8-inch baking pan, parchment paper, medium-large bowl

Prep: 10 minutes
Freeze: 3 hours

1. Line an 8-inch by 8-inch baking pan with parchment paper.

2. In a medium-large bowl, combine all ingredients *except* strawberries. Mix until smooth and uniform.

3. Transfer to the baking pan, and smooth out the top.

4. Top with strawberries, and lightly press to adhere.

5. Cover and freeze until solid, at least 3 hours.

MAKES 6 SERVINGS

PEANUT BUTTER PIE IN A MUG

 Entire recipe: 206 calories, 3.5g total fat (1.5g sat fat), 171mg sodium, 32g carbs, 2g fiber, 20.5g sugars, 11g protein

4

¾ cup **fat-free vanilla yogurt**
1½ tablespoons **powdered peanut butter**
2 tablespoons **natural light whipped topping**
½ sheet (2 crackers) **chocolate graham crackers**, crushed

206 CALORIES

You'll need: mug

Prep: 5 minutes

1. In a mug, thoroughly mix yogurt with powdered peanut butter.

2. Top with whipped topping and crushed graham crackers.

MAKES 1 SERVING

EXTRA, EXTRA!

Top with peanuts for a nutty crunch.

HG TIP

This sweet treat is PERFECT for breakfast!

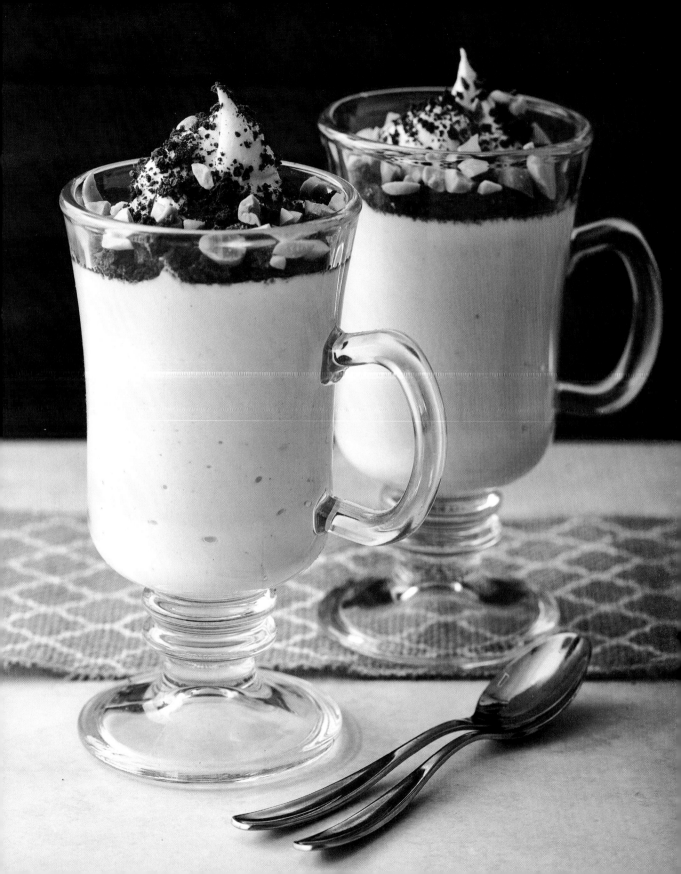

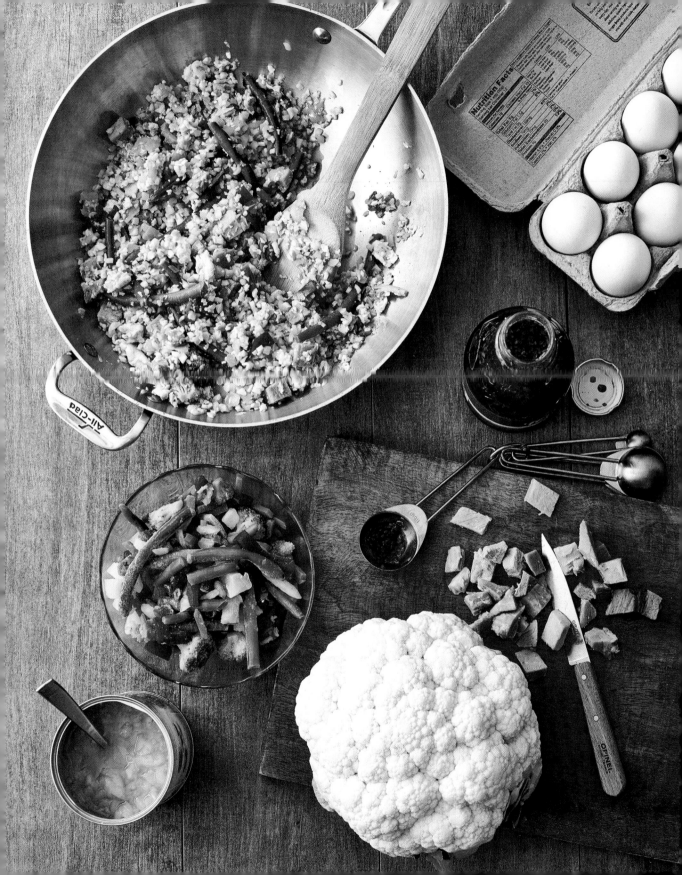

10

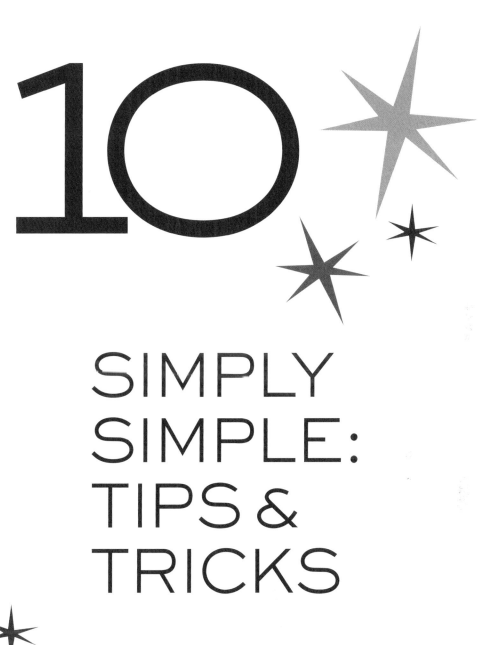

SIMPLY SIMPLE: TIPS & TRICKS

Just when you thought things couldn't get any easier, here's a bonus chapter that's packed with helpful info . . . plus a few pop-up recipes!

Seasonings Made Simple

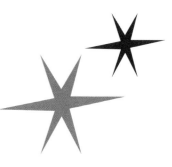

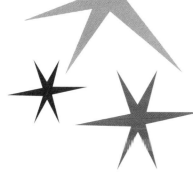

Spices are the ultimate recipe accessory. (Think of them as tasty jewels for your food!) But no need to build an entire arsenal of seasonings in your kitchen.

You can make almost all the recipes in this book with just these basics:

Salt • Black pepper • Garlic powder • Onion powder • Cinnamon • Italian seasoning • Ground cumin • Dried oregano • Chili powder

Ready to kick things up a notch? Stock your spice drawer with taco seasoning, chili seasoning, and everything bagel seasoning! **Or DIY with these simple recipes . . .**

DIY CHILI SEASONING

 ⅒th of recipe (about 1 teaspoon): 5 calories, <0.5g total fat (0g sat fat), 128mg sodium, 1g carbs, 0.5g fiber, <0.5g sugars, <0.5g protein

6

1½ tablespoons **chili powder**
1 teaspoon **ground cumin**
½ teaspoon **garlic powder**
½ teaspoon **salt**
¼ teaspoon **cayenne pepper**
¼ teaspoon **dried oregano**

You'll need: small sealable container

Prep: 5 minutes

1. In a small sealable container, mix ingredients until uniform.

2. Seal and store in a cool dry place.

MAKES 10 SERVINGS

DIY EVERYTHING BAGEL SEASONING

 ⅒th of recipe (about 1 teaspoon): 11 calories, 1g total fat (0g sat fat), 104mg sodium, 0.5g carbs, <0.5g fiber, <0.5g sugars, <0.5g protein

6

1 tablespoon **white sesame seeds**
2 teaspoons **black sesame seeds**
1 teaspoon **dried minced onion**
1 teaspoon **poppy seeds**
1 teaspoon **dried garlic flakes**
½ teaspoon coarse **sea salt**

You'll need: small sealable container

Prep: 5 minutes

1. In a small sealable container, mix ingredients until uniform.

2. Seal and store in a cool dry place.

MAKES 10 SERVINGS

DIY TACO SEASONING

¹⁄₁₀th of recipe (about 1 teaspoon): 9 calories, <0.5g total fat (0g sat fat), 250mg sodium, 1.5g carbs, 0.5g fiber, <0.5g sugars, <0.5g protein

6

2 tablespoons **chili powder**
4 teaspoons **ground cumin**
1 teaspoon **paprika**
1 teaspoon **salt**
½ teaspoon **garlic powder**
½ teaspoon **onion powder**

9 CALORIES

You'll need: small sealable container

Prep: 5 minutes

1. In a small sealable container, mix ingredients until uniform.

2. Seal and store in a cool dry place.

MAKES 10 SERVINGS

USE IT IN . . .

Southwest Muffin-Pan Egg Bakes	53
Sheet-Pan Chicken Fajitas	140
Mexi-licious Zucchini Boats	156
Beefy Cauliflower Rice Stir-Fry	171
Tex-Mex Meatloaf Minis	179
Steak & Avocado Soft Tacos	187
Tropical Fish Tacos	212
Spicy Sofritas Tacos	226
Mexican Cauliflower Rice	251

SODIUM SAVING MADE SIMPLE

I always aim to keep sodium counts in check without sacrificing flavor, but I also know that some people prefer even less sodium in their diets. Here are some simple tips to reduce your salt intake . . .

1. Trade the salt shaker for other flavor boosters.

If you just omit the salt, you'll probably be left craving more flavor! So reach for powerhouse ingredients like lemon juice, lime juice, spices, fresh herbs, and vinegar. If a recipe already contains one or two of these, simply up the amounts.

2. Go for salt-free seasoning mixes.

When a recipe calls for a mix like taco seasoning, grab a no-sodium option like the kind by Mrs. Dash. You can also make the Hungry Girl versions (pages 357–358) without any salt at all. These mixes are even good for seasoning raw protein before cooking, in place of salt and pepper. Bland chicken or flavorless beef is never an acceptable option!

3. Make DIY marinara and salsa.

Jarred sauces and salsas are convenient, but you can save some serious sodium by making them at home. For marinara, simply season up some canned crushed tomatoes with garlic powder, onion powder, and Italian seasoning. To make your own salsa, mix diced tomato and onion with cilantro, jalapeño, lime juice, garlic, and cumin.

4. Cut sodium from canned beans.

Just draining and rinsing canned beans (as called for in Hungry Girl recipes) washes away about 30 percent of the sodium! Reduce the salt count even further by starting with reduced-sodium or even no-salt-added beans. Super simple!

SLOW COOKERS MADE SIMPLE

Slow cookers are super popular, and with good reason!
I love the whole "set it and forget it" approach. For these recipes, you'll want a slow cooker with at least a 6-quart capacity.

No time for a slow-cooked meal, or just don't own a slow cooker?
Use your stove! You can churn out most slow-cooker creations in under an hour . . .

- **Grab a pot with a lid.** You're basically re-creating the slow-cooker environment right on your stove.

- **Set the temperature to medium heat.** You want to simmer the food, not boil it.

- **Start checking on your food at the 35-minute mark.** Your average slow-cooker recipe will be done after 35 to 45 minutes. Easy peasy!

Flip to page 34 to see a list of all the slow-cooker recipes!

INSTANT POT MADE SIMPLE

Ready to cook with the world's coolest kitchen gadget? Here's the need-to-know info . . .

- **The Instant Pot preheats *after* you add your ingredients.** Don't worry . . . That's factored into the total cook time listed with each of these recipes!

- **There will be steam, and it will be HOT.** When you turn the knob to release the burst of steam, I recommend using a towel and then stepping out of the way!

- **You can speed up your favorite slow-cooker recipes by making them in an Instant Pot.** Most slow-cooker dishes will take around 30 minutes to make in your Instant Pot . . . Just use the pressure cooking setting.

- **No Instant Pot? No problem!** A pressure cooker or slow cooker will do the trick. To slow cook, set for 3 to 4 hours on high or 7 to 8 hours on low. If the recipe calls for sautéing, that can be done in a skillet on the stove.

Visit page 34 for a list of all the Instant Pot recipes in this book!

ZUCCHINI NOODLES MADE SIMPLE

Spiralized zucchini is one of my FAVORITE low-calorie, low-carb pasta swaps . . . and it's easier to prepare than you might think!

DIY (Do It Yourself)

What you'll need:
Do yourself a favor, and buy a spiral veggie slicer. Veggetti and OXO make great inexpensive ones (around $10 or so). The fancy tabletop versions are surprisingly affordable as well, but I tend to stick with a standard handheld one. You could use a standard veggie peeler, but a spiralizer will give you the quickest and best results. Spiralized noodles are similar to spaghetti, while zucchini noodles prepped with a peeler is more like fettuccine.

How to make 'em:

- **If you have a spiralizer . . .** Holding the stem end, feed the zucchini into the blade, rotating to churn out the noodles. If your noodles are long, give 'em a rough chop.
- **If you're working with a peeler . . .** Peel the zucchini into thin strips, rotating the zucchini after each swipe of the peeler so that the slices are uniform in size.
- **Make-ahead tip!** Spiralize oodles of zoodles at once, and store them in an airtight container in the fridge. They'll last for days, and you can just break 'em out when you're ready to whip up a dish.

LTDIFY (Let Them Do It for You!)

Look for fresh zucchini noodles in the produce section: Those are recipe ready! Frozen zucchini spirals are another great option . . .

How to use frozen zucchini noodles in recipes . . .
Don't just toss them into the skillet like you would if they were fresh . . . You'll likely end up with a way-too-watery dish. Instead, cook them according to the package direction (for a few minutes in the microwave or a pan on the stove). Then drain them to nix any excess water. Add the noodles for the final minute or so of cook time, just long enough to make sure they're hot and well mixed.

A list of all the zucchini noodle recipes can be found in the index on page 384!

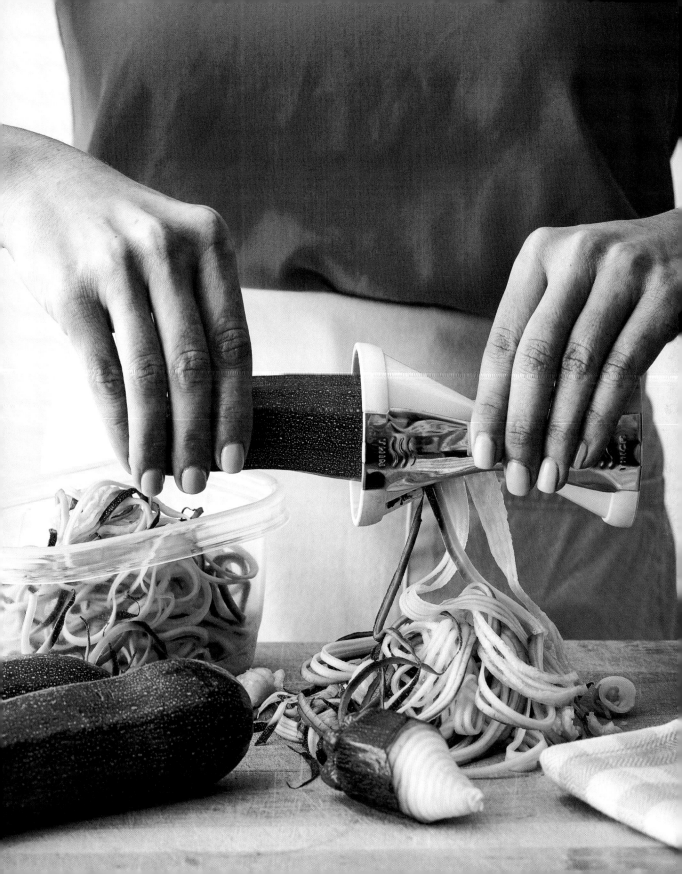

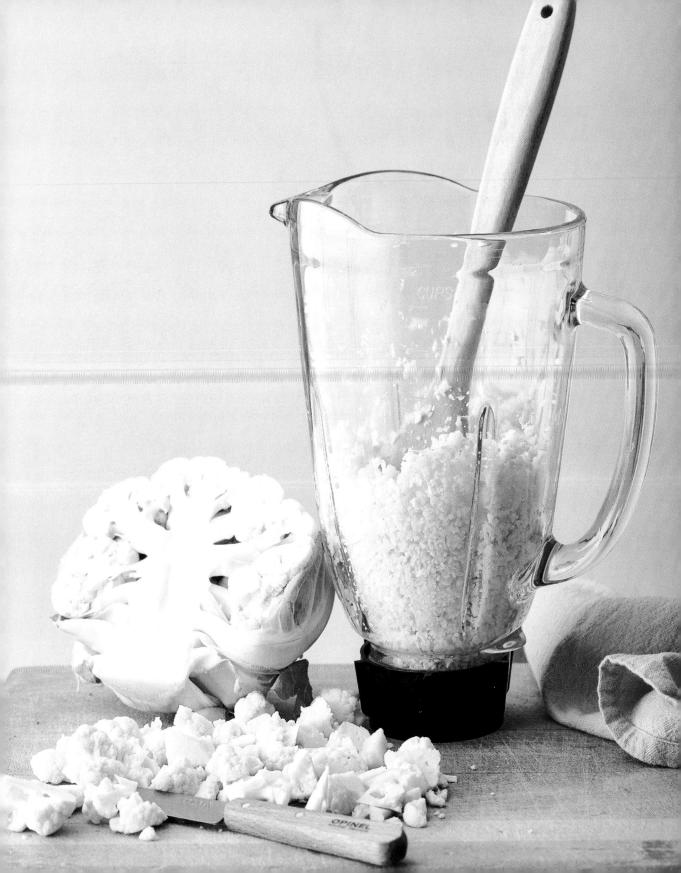

CAULIFLOWER RICE MADE SIMPLE

How did we EXIST before riced cauliflower?! Forget all about traditional calorie-dense rice. Fiber-packed cauliflower rice is here to stay . . .

DIY (Do It Yourself)

What you'll need:
A basic blender is all it takes to blitz the cruciferous vegetable into rice-sized pieces. If you use a food processor, you'll likely end up with crumbs of cauliflower instead. Pass!

How to make it:
The biggest mistake people make when blending cauliflower into rice is starting with florets that are too large. You need nicely chopped cauliflower for your blender to do the job well. Once you've got your chopped veg, pulse it in a blender until reduced to rice-sized pieces. You may need to stop and stir occasionally in order to finish the job. Just rearrange the cauliflower in the blender, and then resume blending.

Make-ahead tip!
Just like zucchini noodles, you can prep a big batch of this starch swap and store it in an airtight container in your fridge. It'll stay fresh for days on end and save you time when you're ready to crank out a recipe!

LTDIFY (Let Them Do It for You!)

These days, it's actually very common to spot fresh cauliflower rice in the produce section of the supermarket. Of course, I like the frozen kind as well . . . Such a smart idea to keep it in the freezer at all times!

How to use frozen riced cauliflower in recipes . . .
Since riced cauliflower thaws quickly and doesn't release as much liquid as zucchini noodles, you can add it to your dish at the same time the fresh cauliflower is called for . . . Or just pop it in the microwave per the package directions, and add it to your dish just before serving!

Flip to cauliflower rice in the index to see all the recipes!

MAKE-AHEAD MADE SIMPLE

We're all super busy, and make-ahead meals are crucial for crazed days. When you have some extra time, cook up some of the amazing recipes in this book, and store them in the fridge or freezer. SO many recipes here are ideal make-ahead meals! And these pointers will help make things even easier . . .

Step 1: Prepare the recipe as directed, but leave off any fresh toppings.

Salsa, sour cream, whipped cream, herbs . . . These things are best left for day-of topping off. Just don't forget about 'em altogether. (That would be sad!)

Step 2: Divide and cool.

Divide the dish into equally sized servings, using microwave-safe containers with airtight lids. This way, you'll have perfect portions that cool quickly, thaw nicely, and reheat in no time. If you plan on freezing the meals, look for freezer-friendly containers. For individual items like muffins and mini meatloaves, avoid freezer burn by wrapping them individually once cool; then place them all in a sealable bag or container.

Step 3: Into the fridge or freezer.

Almost ALL the recipes in this book can be refrigerated and will stay fresh for several days. For the DOs and DON'Ts of freezing, see the following page.

Step 4: Reheat and eat!

Make-ahead meals from the fridge are a breeze to prepare. Remove the lid or vent it before placing the container in the microwave. Then heat the dish for a minute at a time (less for smaller items), until it reaches your desired temperature. As for frozen dishes? Flip the page for more!

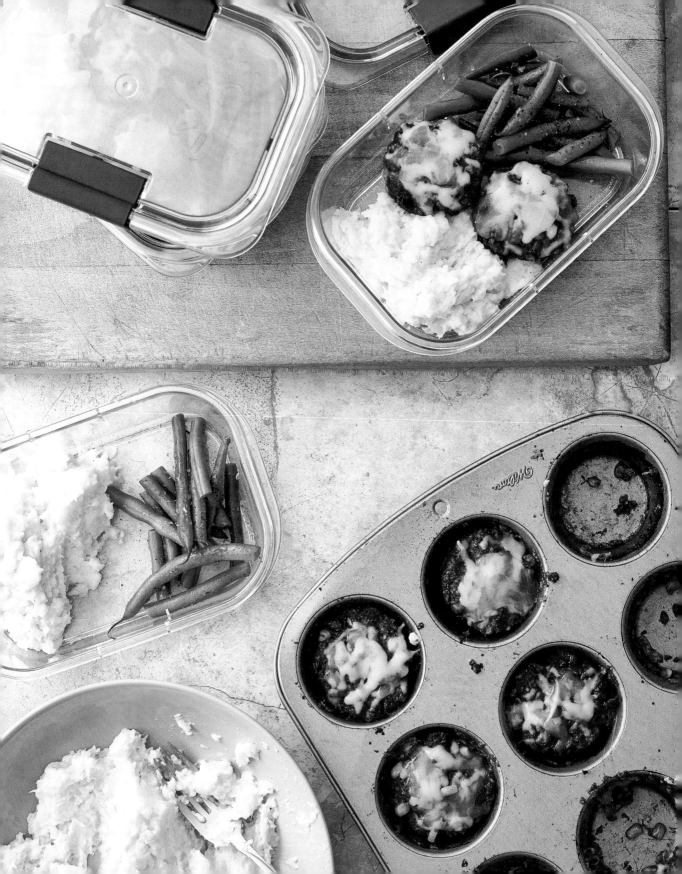

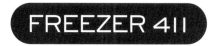

FREEZER 411

Best way to prep . . .

Thaw the dish in the fridge overnight, and simply reheat when you're ready to eat.

Freezer to plate . . .

If you're strapped for time, thaw your food in the microwave using the defrost setting. Check on it every minute or two (less for smaller items), giving it a stir or rotating as needed. Don't forget to unwrap anything sealed in plastic.

What to Freeze

Baked Goods • Soup/Stew • Stir-Frys • Meatloaf • Casseroles • Baked Chicken or Fish • Burger Patties • Meatballs

What NOT to Freeze

The texture of these foods is compromised once thawed and reheated . . .

Hard-Boiled Eggs • Breaded Dishes • Spaghetti Squash • Zucchini Noodles • Dips • Fries

See page 32 for a list of multi-serving recipes . . . perfect for make-ahead meals!

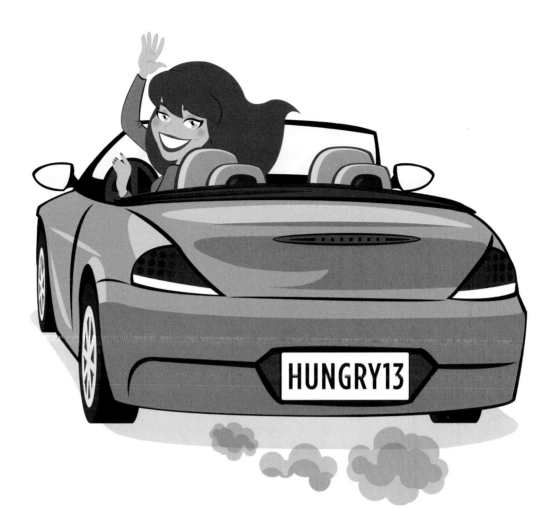

And there they are! Some of the easiest and most delicious recipes EVER. I am completely in love with every single one, and I hope you will be too! For more healthy recipes — plus food finds, tips 'n tricks, and more — sign up for the free daily emails at hungry-girl.com.

'Til next time . . . Chew the right thing!

Lisa :)

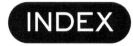

INDEX